Desirée Ciambrone, PhD

Women's Experiences with HIV/AIDS
Mending Fractured Selves

Pre-publication
REVIEW . . .

"**W**omen's Experiences with HIV/ AIDS helps scholars see the contributions that a really good qualitative study can make to a body of knowledge. Dr. Ciambrone has meticulously detailed the lives of the women in her study; the reader has the sense of being a silent observer of their lives. Using Bury's theory of repair of disrupted biographies, she helps the reader understand the complexity of the women's lives. Dr. Ciambrone casts an unflinching eye on her subjects, letting the reader see them as the complex, fasci-nating women that they are. The result is a rich tapestry woven from the women's narratives and the existing literature on women with HIV. This book makes a significant contribution to our knowledge of women and HIV, and to qualitative research."

Julie Barroso, PhD, ANP, CS
Assistant Professor,
University of North Carolina
School of Nursing,
Chapel Hill

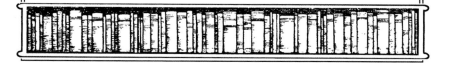

Women's Experiences with HIV/AIDS

Mending Fractured Selves

HAWORTH Psychosocial Issues of HIV/AIDS
R. Dennis Shelby, PhD
Senior Editor

Women's Experiences with HIV/AIDS
Mending Fractured Selves

Desirée Ciambrone, PhD

The Haworth Press®
New York • London • Oxford

The Haworth Press, Inc., 10 Alice Street, Binghamton, NY 13904-1580.

PUBLISHER'S NOTE: To ensure the anonymity of interviewees, pseudonyms are used for respondents' names.

Cover design by Lora Wiggins.

Library of Congress Cataloging-in-Publication Data

Ciambrone, Desirée
  Women's experiences with HIV/AIDS : mending fractured selves / Desirée Ciambrone.
    p. cm.
  Includes bibliographical references and index.
  ISBN 0-7890-1757-1 (alk. paper)—ISBN 0-7890-1758-X (soft)
    1. AIDS (Disease) in women—Psychological aspects. 2. AIDS (Disease) in women—Social aspects. I. Title.

RC606.6 .C535 2003
362.1'969792'0082—dc21

2002068756

For my mother, Dolores Maiello Ciambrone,
and in loving memory of my father,
William F. Ciambrone

ABOUT THE AUTHOR

Desirée Ciambrone, PhD, is an Agency for Healthcare Research and Quality postdoctoral fellow at the Center for Gerontology and Health Care Research at Brown University in Providence, Rhode Island. Her interests include medical sociology, women's health, disability, psychosocial adjustment to chronic illness, and informal care giving/social support. She has done research focusing on spousal support among women with illness and the psychosocial sequelae among breast cancer survivors. As a qualitative medical sociologist, Dr. Ciambrone has researched a variety of populations, including women with HIV/AIDS, adults with mental retardation, adults with mental illness, and young adults who returned home to live with their parents. Dr. Ciambrone has co-authored several articles investigating how individuals cope with illness, published in journals including *Research on Aging, Sociology of Health & Illness,* and *The Gerontologist.*

CONTENTS

Acknowledgments

Many people provided support and direction in the preparation of this manuscript. I would like to thank Phil Brown, my dissertation chair, for his mentoring and encouragement throughout my graduate studies and postgraduate work. Susan Allen was also a constant source of support and guidance. I thank her for her intellectual contribution to this research and for her continued mentoring and friendship. The valuable comments and suggestions given by Ann Dill and Lynn Davidman also helped to shape this project, particularly during its earliest stages.

My friends and colleagues have also been a tremendous source of encouragement in the course of conducting this study. I especially want to thank Gaelan Benway, Lori Hunter, Voon Chin Phua, Lisa Welch, Esther Wilder, and Susan Zimmermann. I am very grateful to my friends and colleagues at the Center for Gerontology and Health Care Research for providing the support necessary for the completion of this book.

I owe a special note of thanks to my mother, Dolores Maiello Ciambrone, for her unwavering support, and to my sister, Darlene Ciambrone, who painstakingly transcribed each of my interviews. I am also grateful to my husband, Edward Simpson, for his companionship and interest in my work.

I extend my gratitude to the many individuals who introduced me to the interviewees.

Finally, this study would not have been possible without the cooperation of the women I interviewed. I am deeply grateful to them for welcoming me into their lives and sharing their stories with me.

Chapter 1

Introduction

DISRUPTION AND LEGITIMATION: HILLARY

Hillary is a fifty-four-year-old, heavyset woman with fair skin. She is a vivacious, candid woman who is as articulate as she is humorous; she also has acquired immunodeficiency syndrome (AIDS). Hillary works as a ministry outreach worker for disadvantaged community members. As part of her work she refers marginalized people with human immunodeficiency virus (HIV) and AIDS to appropriate social and medical services. Hillary's work is dear to her heart, and it helps her cope with her own illness.

Prior to 1988, Hillary led a happy life. As a youngster, she was a good student and got along well with her parents. After she graduated from high school she got married and had two children. She divorced in 1979 and derived satisfaction from her job in the service sector and from her young-adult children.

Within a year or two, Hillary met her second husband, Charles. Charles was open with Hillary about his heroin addiction and explained that he had been clean for only two months prior to their meeting. In the late 1970s, AIDS was the farthest thing from Hillary's mind, and when the couple started to engage in sexual relations, she used an intrauterine device (IUD) instead of condoms to protect against pregnancy. In 1988 her husband was diagnosed with AIDS. Charles' sickness shattered Hillary's world:

> My life before HIV and AIDS was people's normal lives. I had a good marriage the second time around. I had a good relationship with my children. . . . We just thought we had everything. I mean we weren't well off or anything, but we made it financially. And we had a lot of love and a lot of laughter. . . . He was my best friend as well as my husband. And so when that happened it was like my world was never the same.

Shortly after Charles, in 1988, Hillary also received her seropositive diagnosis. Given that she and her husband had not protected themselves from sexually transmitted diseases, Hillary's diagnosis was not a surprise. Their sickness, however, disrupted Hillary's life and future plans. Former familiar ways of thinking about her life as well as her behavior demanded reorganization. Further, HIV/AIDS altered the ways in which she perceived herself relative to other people. Hillary had been a happy, confident woman, but when she found out that she was HIV positive, she felt "dirty" and inferior. She felt "less than anybody else . . . because of the stigma of the disease."

While devotedly caring for Charles until his death in 1991, Hillary did not have time or energy to tend to her own well-being. After he died she turned her attention to her own physical and emotional health. Despite her vigilance, in 1995 Hillary's health deteriorated and she was diagnosed with AIDS. Hillary continues to take her antiretroviral medication faithfully, wearing a pager to ensure she does not forget to take her pills; she is well aware that missing dosages, even sporadically, can markedly interfere with the effectiveness of the medication. In addition, Hillary eats nutritious foods and abstains from alcohol and other known health risks. Further, although Hillary was not involved in an intimate relationship at the time of her interview, she has always informed her sexual partners of her status and has always insisted on practicing safe sex since she contracted HIV.

Hillary discussed living with HIV/AIDS in terms of death, deterioration, and changes in physical appearance. She is not afraid of death. In fact, in her work as a client advocate for disadvantaged people with HIV/AIDS, she stresses the need for candor when dealing with death. Despite her acceptance and openness about death, however, she is not immune to the social construction of femininity with its concomitant emphasis on physical appearance—that which illness compromises and, at worst, destroys. Hillary articulately discussed her concern, cognizant of the pressure on women to conform to cultural standards of beauty:

> For me, losing my looks is a big concern. And it shouldn't be that important compared to losing your life or your ability to be self-sufficient, but I've seen what it does to you, and it's a scary thing. Dying doesn't scare me; losing my looks scares me. [Women] are valued on our looks, you know, and so that's a big concern for me.

Despite her fear of a painful AIDS-related death, in the eight years since Hillary was diagnosed she has coped well with her illness. Relational resources have been central to Hillary's incorporation of HIV into her life. Her children's acceptance and support has been a critical resource. She and her adult son and daughter share an open, loving relationship. They fully support her activist work and are in close contact with Hillary.

Hillary's activist work is also one of her primary coping strategies. In addition to her ministry work, Hillary is a volunteer AIDS activist/educator and a prison HIV/AIDS support group facilitator. In terms of living and coping with AIDS, this involvement has helped her tremendously. For years Hillary remained silent because her husband preferred that no one know of his serostatus, including his family. When she was able to disclose her diagnosis, it was "the best thing, it was an incredibly freeing experience." For years now, Hillary has been in the public eye doing local television news appearances and sharing her story. Hillary clearly has made personal gains from her activist work. Beyond helping herself cope with AIDS, she acts on behalf of all women with HIV and in so doing reframes her identity in positive terms:

> In fact, sometimes I'm almost proud of the fact that I have it. And that sounds strange; I don't really know how to put it in the right words, but it's like here I am, I have this, I'm well with my life. I do good things; I'm a good person; I dare you to say something [bad about] me.

Hillary's work does, at times, take a toll on her health. She often has to remind herself to take time off for bed rest. Despite the exhaustion, Hillary feels that the psychosocial benefits she receives from her work far outweigh potential health detriments. In fact, she enthusiastically articulated the impact of her psychosocial well-being on her physical health:

> I can't stop sometimes so I just push myself to keep going. . . . I do a lot. But that's my way of living with my disease and giving something back, and feeling like what's left of my life isn't a waste. And I love what I do. . . . It makes me tired, but it makes me healthier because I love it and I don't sit home feeling sorry for myself and dwelling on my disease.

Thus, Hillary has a realistic view of her illness and its severity, and she is able to point out the ways in which HIV has had positive consequences in her life. "I don't cry about it all the time, but you wake up with it and you go to sleep with it and it's always a part of your life, and for me, more positive things have come out of it than negative things. It's made me a better person. . . . I know I'm as good as anybody else even with this disease and I know I have a lot to offer."

Hillary is well aware of the typical AIDS downward illness trajectory. She knows that although antiretroviral therapy may slow down disease progression, as yet there is no cure for AIDS. By taking care of herself, enjoying her family, and actively occupying her time with social service work, she is living with AIDS as best she can. Her life has been deeply disrupted by the disease, yet she continually seeks to legitimize many components of her life. In her attempt to find strength, wholeness, and self-respect, Hillary is engaging in the "repair" of her "disrupted biography" (Bury 1982). Hillary is a rather successful example of repair work.

PROBLEMATIC REPAIR STRATEGIES: DENISE

Denise was interviewed nearly a month after Hillary, in 1996. The meeting took place in her mother's home where she resides with her adolescent daughter and son. They live in their small, cluttered home in a low-income neighborhood. Never married, Denise has lived with her mother for the past twenty-four years, but has often left home during her drug-using years and for participation in rehabilitation programs. Denise has been using marijuana and cocaine since she was thirteen years old and has experimented with intravenous drugs. At age thirty-eight, Denise looked much older than her age. Her lifestyle and hardships showed on her face; she looked weary and unkempt. When Denise was younger she worked in a factory, but she has not worked outside the home in over ten years. As a result of her drug use and social isolation, Denise does not have a strong friendship network and has little contact with people outside of her immediate family.

Despite the fact that Denise has had to contend with other hardships, she describes HIV as a very disruptive event. When she received her test results she felt desperate and suicidal. She compared this to the period just prior to receiving her diagnosis and said that she was an "outgoing, happy-go-lucky person." Denise had curbed her cocaine use and turned to marijuana instead. Perceiving this as good progress, her diagnosis threatened her improvement. In fact, Denise had been clean only about two months at the time of the meeting. Despite her drug use, she considered herself to be "normal," and HIV infection to represent that which is "abnormal." Although she has had unprotected sex with multiple partners who were also drug users, she strongly believes that she contracted HIV as a result of being raped by a man she knew who "just flipped out." When told she was HIV positive, Denise acted out and "tried to destroy [the ladies' rest room], tried to take that toilet off the floor." Feeling as if she had received a death sentence, she contemplated suicide and began smoking cocaine again. "I said, 'Okay, I'm gonna die,' couldn't deal with it, and I didn't understand too much about it. So I just started doing a lot of drugs and tried to not deal with that."

Denise admits that she tries not to acknowledge her illness. On the other hand, she claims she is not in denial. As she said, "I let people know, you know—not that I *have* to, it's just that's just how I am, that's how I deal with my sickness . . . by lettin' people know." By people, Denise is referring primarily to her immediate kin whom she credits with providing emotional support. "They still love me. They're there for me. [When] I have my sad, blue days, they're there for me." Denise has little contact with those outside of her familial and health care provider networks. She has never attended a support group for people with HIV/AIDS and said, "the only support group I have is my family."

Denise no longer perceives HIV as a great threat to her health because her T-cell count has remained above critical levels and she has not used drugs for a couple of months. Living with HIV for nearly seven years prior to this study, Denise has reconstructed HIV into a minor problem and sees her drug addiction as most problematic. She feels that if she can remain clean her health will be fine: "I'm glad I [am] just staying off those drugs. I just stay in the house. I see my [family] and that's it. . . . But just thank God I don't do the things I used to do. I feel a lot better. . . . I can think, I can function, you know what I'm saying? I don't snap at my mother; I don't snap at people."

In contrast to Hillary, Denise has an unrealistic view of the virus. She believes that because she is off drugs, HIV will not pose any serious problems. In fact, she does not worry about the welfare of her children should she become ill or functionally impaired because she feels she will outlive them: "It doesn't bother me 'cause I can live probably longer than they [will]. See, because what the cocaine does, it progresses the virus; it breaks the body down; it just kills the immune system. But now that I'm drug free, I don't worry about nothin' anymore."

Denise's drug use undoubtedly posed a great threat to her already compromised health, and staying clean is a crucial factor in successful HIV/AIDS treatment. Abstaining from illicit drugs alone, however, is not a cure, and there is no guarantee that she will not become symptomatic or progress to full-blown AIDS. In fact, the chances are great that her health will become progressively worse as time passes. Thus, Denise may be less likely to comply with drug therapies or worry about infecting others. Although Denise takes her medications and gets regular medical checkups, she does not practice safe sex. Further, by ignoring or downplaying the effects of HIV on her health, she may be ill prepared to deal with the psychosocial effects of deterioration and dying.

Denise's narrative is full of contradictions. For example, she said she is coping well with HIV by being open about her illness, but has not told many others about her diagnosis. She has not engaged in any vehicles to promote disclosure, such as support groups. She views HIV/AIDS as a "death sentence," but is largely unconcerned with practicing safe sex. She is also much less articulate than Hillary and other respondents in this study. She provided fewer details about her experiences and was unable to provide a great deal of specific background information, particularly in regard to her life prior to contracting HIV. Many of the women in this sample were more articulate and active in AIDS-related projects than Denise. However, it is important to listen to the stories of women such as Denise, as she is probably representative of many of the women infected with HIV/AIDS, women whose efforts at repairing disrupted biographies are only partially successful.

DISRUPTION AND NONREPAIR: STEPHANIE

Stephanie is thirty-eight years old and had been living with HIV infection for eight years at the time of the study. She never married and has no children. She lives in a beautiful, spacious home with her sister and brother-in-law in a middle-class Northeastern suburb. Stephanie lost her mother when she was seventeen years old and her relationship with her father has always been strained. Her father denied her mother's mental illness and refused to take responsibility for abusing his wife and children. In addition, Stephanie was sexually molested by a family member. In an attempt to break away from her family, Stephanie joined the military and was trained as an electronics technician. Due to a drop in her T-cell count and increasing stress, she recently stopped working and has started taking courses at a nearby university.

Prior to contracting HIV infection, Stephanie was involved in an unfulfilling romantic relationship and was battling depression. Stephanie does not have a drug use history, but decided to be tested because she had dated a heroin addict and knew the risks associated with sharing needles. Prior to receiving her diagnosis, she had "read a few articles and stuff like that" and was familiar with the modes of HIV transmission. In addition, her most recent lover had apparently engaged in risky behavior. Although he never divulged the exact nature of his actions, Stephanie suspects he may have either experimented with intravenous drugs or had a "one-night stand."

Although Stephanie went for testing because "it seemed like the right thing to do," she was confident that the results would come back negative: "I really didn't really believe that it would happen. It's just denial, you know?" Upon receiving her diagnosis Stephanie was retested two more times, just in case they were false-positive results.

Despite Stephanie's efforts to ignore her condition, she got the flu shortly after her diagnosis and was forced to acknowledge her illness. She is open about the fact that she has still not come to terms with having HIV/AIDS. For Stephanie, one of the most disruptive aspects of HIV/AIDS is the concomitant stigma and discrimination. To avoid being stigmatized, Stephanie does not form new close ties. Her fear of being ostracized is particularly problematic because she wants very much to be romantically involved. Despite her desire, however, she is afraid of disclosing her seropositivity for fear of rejection. During the interview, Stephanie spent a good deal of time discussing her apprehension. She explained that having to disclose her status presents a barrier to dating:

It's really hard because if I was going to be involved with someone I'd have to tell them I was HIV positive. . . . To tell someone,
that is like a really big thing, you know? . . . I've been really
cautious—maybe overly cautious because even when it's kind
of obvious that people probably wouldn't hold it against you,
you still feel like well, even if they still want to be your friends,
maybe they'll be afraid . . . because the fear is so great.

In addition, Stephanie would very much like to have children, but
feels that the risk of giving birth to an HIV-positive infant outweighs
her longing to be a mother; thus, the disruption associated with her
illness is particularly severe. Because Stephanie was only beginning
to work HIV into her biography, discussing her illness was a very
painful experience. In fact, Stephanie was the only woman who became so upset during our conversation that she broke down in tears.

Relative to other respondents, Stephanie is having a very difficult
time dealing with the multiple losses associated with HIV/AIDS as
well as working the illness into her biography. Despite Stephanie's
abusive childhood, in discussing how each of these events altered her
biography and sense of self, she concentrated on sickness and the fatal nature of HIV/AIDS. She described HIV infection as the most disruptive event in her life "because it's life threatening":

I mean [HIV] was the biggest thing. . . . There is a lot of denial
still for a really long time where I felt . . . more optimistic and
felt more hopeful like, "I know I'm gonna survive and they're
gonna find something before anything happens to me, you
know?" But that's denial to a degree, too. But now it's a lot
harder, since I had the low count . . . it's becoming a lot more real
for me these days because having been just a little bit sick . . . just
enough to put a good scare into me.

HIV/AIDS prompted Stephanie to seek counseling. Although therapy has helped Stephanie come to grips with her dysfunctional family
and the silence surrounding her mother's illness, it has been less successful in helping her cope with HIV infection. She has also turned to
support groups, but has been unable to derive much consolation from
them. Stephanie has a hard time connecting with other women with
HIV/AIDS due to her higher socioeconomic class and lifestyle differ-

ences (e.g., no history of drug use). Of her experiences in support groups, Stephanie said:

> I always felt like I didn't have anything to complain about when I looked at the other people. They weren't supportive for me because I would always go in there and feel like my problems were small because the other people were really sick, or really impoverished, or having these huge problems and, you know, I had a job and plenty of money. I had excellent health care, I was fine physically, so I didn't really connect with the people that well.

She continues to look for other avenues to foster repair.

For Stephanie, HIV/AIDS has caused a great disruption that is not easy to fix. With the strong emotional support she receives from her sister, Stephanie is trying to lead a normal life. In an effort to combat illness progression, Stephanie takes good care of herself and adheres to her treatment regimen. However, in contrast to many of the women in this study, HIV constantly occupies Stephanie's thoughts and she has been largely unable to reconstruct a positive identity. Although many women have pointed out the negative *and* positive effects of their illness, Stephanie does not see any positive consequences resulting from HIV infection. She is having an extremely difficult time repairing her disrupted biography.

* * *

The following chapters tell of women similar to Hillary, Denise, and Stephanie; women who appear to be adjusting well to HIV/AIDS, and women who do not appear to be adjusting well to their illness; women who have adopted beneficial coping strategies, and women who have adopted problematic styles of coping; women who are protecting themselves from further decline, and others from infection; and women who are less concerned with self-care and virus transmission.

HIV/AIDS AS A GENDER ISSUE

Women comprise the fastest-growing subgroup of the HIV population in the United States and approximately 20 percent of those living with AIDS (Kaiser Foundation 2001). Over a thirteen-year period the proportion of AIDS cases among women has more than tripled, from 7 percent in 1985 to 23 percent in 1999 (CDC 1999).

The initial recognition of HIV/AIDS as a gay male disease has been particularly consequential for women. Considering women to be a low-risk group, medical professionals have often attributed their symptoms to problems less serious than HIV infection (Shayne and Kaplan 1991). Moreover, the definition of AIDS, prior to its redefinition in 1993, failed to include gynecologic symptoms commonly associated with HIV infection in women, such as increased incidence of pelvic inflammatory disease, cervical cancer, and severe, persistent vaginal yeast infections (Bury 1995; Lather and Smithies 1997; Rosser 1991). The lack of a clear understanding of the etiology of the disease in women has led to underdiagnosis and misdiagnosis of cases among women (Corea 1992; Kaspar 1989; Rodriguez-Trias and Marte 1995; Scharf 1992; Weitz 1993; Smeltzer and Whipple 1991).

Women are biologically and socially more vulnerable to HIV infection than their male counterparts (Bury 1995; Corea 1992; Crystal and Sambamoorthi 1996; Hellinger 1993; Kaspar 1989; Rodriguez-Trias and Marte 1995; Scharf 1992; Weitz 1993; Shayne and Kaplan 1991; Lather and Smithies 1997; Rosser 1991). Male-to-female transmission, for example, is more efficient than female-to-male transmission (Crystal and Sambamoorthi 1996; Lather and Smithies 1997; Persson 1994). Women with HIV infection are more likely to be victims of domestic violence and are more likely to lack financial support (Flanigan 1995). Women's lack of power and their dependence on men may make it extremely difficult or even impossible to negotiate safe sex via condom use (Crystal and Sambamoorthi 1996; Fullilove et al. 1990; Holland et al. 1990). Women with HIV may have trouble dealing with the health care system due to functional impairments, low incomes, transportation difficulties, and multiple caregiving responsibilities (Crystal and Sambamoorthi 1996). Furthermore, women generally lack the political organization and support that gay men have garnered (Campbell 1990; Friedman et al. 1992; Schneider 1992; Suffet and Lifshitz 1991; Ward 1993).

This lack of social power reflects the social place of most women with HIV/AIDS. Marginalized women are overrepresented among women with HIV/AIDS; HIV-infected women tend to be poor, nonwhite, and intravenous (IV) drug users (Schneider and Stoller 1995;

Shayne and Kaplan 1991; Weitz 1993). Typically, women of color are at a distinct disadvantage due to scarce economic resources and greater barriers to health and social services (Ward 1993). In addition, they are more likely to be victims of domestic violence and racial discrimination (Bradley-Springer 1994; Flanigan 1995).

Research also suggests that women with HIV/AIDS suffer multiple losses, including the loss of loved ones, their health, future aspirations, body image, sexuality, childbearing, and financial resources (Henderson 1992; Sherr et al. 1993; Stuntzer-Gibson 1991; Weitz 1990; Wiener 1991). In addition, they experience fear, isolation, and uncertainty (Brander and Norton 1993; Coward 1994), which are heightened by the likelihood of abandonment (Kaspar 1989; Weitz 1993). HIV/AIDS is laden with stigma and fear, which affect self-image and perhaps also available sources of support (Bunting 2001; Conrad 1987; Crystal and Schiller 1993; Wiener 1991).

These issues are often compounded by women's responsibility for the domestic sphere (Chung and Magraw 1992). Women who are ill are often expected to care for others while simultaneously tending to their own health, which places many women in a position of triple jeopardy; that is, they are dealing with their own infection, worrying about possible infection of their children, as well as looking after other people with HIV/AIDS (Campbell 1990; Dowling 1995; Hackl et al. 1997; Rodriguez-Trias and Marte 1995; Schneider and Stoller 1995; Ward 1993). Having primary responsibility for household labor and child care often leaves HIV-positive women with little time to engage in self-care activities (e.g., getting proper rest and exercise), and may prevent them from seeking medical treatment (ACT UP 1990; Flanigan 1995).

Women's domestic burdens may well contribute to HIV-related stressors such as poverty, physical impairment, and psychological distress. On the other hand, given the centrality of caring in women's lives, the inability to continue nurturing, due to sickness or other circumstances, may negatively affect self-esteem and facilitate biographical disruption (Lamping and Mercey 1996; Lea 1994; Melvin 1996). Faced with an uncertain illness characterized by a loss of control, caring labor may well serve as an important coping mechanism and way to preserve a sense of self threatened by chronic illness (Charmaz 1991; Pivnick 1994).

* * *

This interview-based study explores the effects of HIV/AIDS on women's daily lives. It looks at how women with HIV give meaning to their illness experience—how they talk about and describe the impact of the illness on their lives and the ways in which the disease is linked to broader social constructions (e.g., gender) and institutions (e.g., health care and social services). Given the unique place of women in the AIDS epidemic, this book addresses the following research questions: How does HIV infection affect women's sense of self? In the face of a stigmatizing illness, how do women repair disruption and restore identities? What are the limits to women's coping strategies? Will these strategies work if women become functionally impaired or develop AIDS? How do women's structural and social environments facilitate or impede repair? What role do women's informal networks play in biographical disruption and repair work?

ANALYTIC FRAMEWORK: BIOGRAPHICAL DISRUPTION AND HIV/AIDS

In order to address these questions, this text will draw from social science literature (e.g., sociological, psychological, social work, and nursing) regarding chronic illness, coping, social support, and gender. Researchers within these fields who highlight the impact of chronic illness on identity as well as the actions individuals take to manage illness (e.g., Bury 1982; Charmaz 1991, 1994; Corbin and Strauss 1988; Kleinman 1988; Robinson 1990; Weitz 1990; Williams 1984) have paved the way for a deeper understanding and greater appreciation of the patient perspective (Brown 1991; Conrad 1987). Concepts derived from this perspective (e.g., stigma, biographical disruption, identity reconstruction, and illness trajectory) have proved invaluable to the study of chronic illness (Bury 1982; Charmaz 1987; Corbin and Strauss 1987; Goffman 1963; Schneider and Conrad 1980).

Crises and traumatic events typically rupture people's lives and affect the ways in which they see themselves. Familiar understandings are threatened or destroyed, and individuals must alter or abandon prior meaning systems to account for novel experiences. Illness is one such event that disrupts lives, and it often demands structural reorganization as well as cognitive restructuring. In times of illness, one's biography or the "who I am at any point along the biographical time line" (Corbin and Strauss 1987: 253) is threatened or altered.

Theoretically, HIV/AIDS represents a severely disruptive event. HIV/AIDS disproportionately affects marginalized, "deviant" groups such as homosexuals and drug users. People with AIDS face considerable stigma and blame for their illness and are often deemed a group unworthy of support. Despite relatively successful recent advances in highly active antiretroviral therapy, there is no cure for AIDS.

In order to describe how women interpret, experience, and subsequently cope with HIV/AIDS, this book will analyze women's narratives in terms of Bury's concepts of biographical disruption and legitimation. Following Strauss and Glaser (1975), Bury (1982) treats chronic illness as a disruptive experience wherein everyday life and fundamental belief systems are disrupted. Biographical disruption includes the disruption of one's former assumptions and behaviors, changes in one's self-concept, and the mobilization of helping networks. Bury distinguishes two subjective meanings of chronic illness as biographical disruption. First, there is the meaning of illness that lies in its consequences, e.g., symptoms and the impact of illness on managing a home and social life. Second, there is significance in terms of the symbolic connotations attached to one's condition (Bury 1982). Due to the stigma associated with HIV/AIDS, we may expect women with HIV infection to report feelings of stigmatization and perhaps a loss of control over certain aspects of their lives.

Dealing with disruption involves biographical work or legitimation. Biographical work may be viewed as a "script for putting one's life back together" (Siegel and Krauss 1991:28), which involves reviewing and reconstructing one's sense of personal and social place. It is through biographical work that chronically ill people regain control of their lives (Siegel and Krauss 1991). According to Bury, disrupted biographies are mended via reconstruction work or "legitimation." Legitimation refers to the ways in which individuals attempt to repair disrupted biographies by "establish[ing] an acceptable and legitimate place for the condition within the person's life . . . [it is an] attempt to maintain a sense of personal integrity, and reduce the threat to social status, in the face of radically altered circumstances" (1991:456). Material, relational, and/or cognitive resources are tapped in the process of repair work.

Analyzing the data within a biographical disruption framework underscores my emphasis on the effects of the illness on women's identities, the meanings women assign to HIV infection, and the ways in which they integrate HIV into their biographies. Although the theory has been applied to men's experiences with HIV/AIDS (see Carricaburu and Pierret 1995), we do not have a clear understanding of how this model reflects women's experiences. Factors including socioeconomic class, sexual preference, and lifestyle differences (e.g., drug use histories) differentially impact individual experiences of health and illness. Thus, although it informs this analysis, the literature on men with HIV/AIDS cannot be extrapolated to HIV-positive women. Further, by analyzing HIV-positive women's experiences of disruption and repair we may gain insight into the practical implications or public health ramifications of their conceptions of, and responses to, illness.

SAMPLE AND METHODOLOGY

From June 1996 to June 1998 thirty-seven HIV-positive women located primarily in the Northeast were interviewed. (Four of the women lived in the South.)

The Appendix provides a demographic summary of the sample discussed in this book. Respondents range in age from twenty-seven to sixty, with a mean age of forty. Twenty-three (62 percent) of the women interviewed identified themselves as white, eleven (30 percent) as black, and three (8 percent) as Latina. The majority were either separated or divorced ($n = 18$, or 49 percent) or never married ($n = 14$, or 38 percent). Only three women were married (8 percent) and two women were widowed (5 percent). As is typical of this population, most (57 percent) had only a high school education/GED or less. Nine women, however, did report having "some college," eight had an associate's degree or professional/trade certification, and two women graduated from a four-year college. Women's annual income ranged from $900 to $40,000, with a mean of $11,084. Most women (62 percent) were not working at the time of the interview.

Nearly 60 percent ($n = 22$) reported contracting the virus via heterosexual sex, slightly fewer from intravenous drug use (IVDU) (32 percent, $n = 12$). Two respondents became infected by ways atypical in the present sample: one woman who did have an IVDU history reported becoming infected by an acquaintance who maliciously stuck her with an infected needle, and another woman was raped by a man carrying the virus. The length of time women had been living with HIV infection ranged from two to thirteen years, with the average being seven years. Five women in the sample were diagnosed with AIDS at the time of the survey.

Women were recruited from diverse agencies serving people with AIDS, including AIDS organizations, drug treatment centers, health clinics, and local drop-in centers for people with AIDS. In seeking a heterogeneous sample, nearly seventy agencies were contacted. Despite such diverse recruitment efforts, however, most of the respondents were referred by a few key contacts. This is due in part to the fact that the many women in Rhode Island and southeastern Massachusetts are already part of a large epidemiological research study. Thus, as a convenience sample, it contains several biases. First, for the most part, the women were well linked in the health care network. Respondents' participation in other area epidemiological studies has provided them with coordinated medical and social services. Thus, overall, these women cannot speak to issues of unmet health and service need, a prevalent problem among women with HIV/AIDS. Similarly, relative to other HIV-positive women, respondents enrolled in this epidemiological study have more experience discussing their wants and needs and are ostensibly more skilled in articulating their stories. Thus, the sample overrepresents women who are attracted to, and experienced in, participation in HIV-related research projects. Findings based on this self-selected group of HIV-positive women may be less applicable to women in other regions who have not received the benefits of participation in a well-organized health care system. Second, despite attempts to oversample women of color, this sample is primarily white. In 1999, African-American women represented 13 percent of the population yet they accounted for 63 percent of newly reported AIDS cases (Kaiser Foundation 2001). Thus, although African-American and Latina women represent less than one-fourth of the U.S. female population, they account for more than three-fourths (76 percent) of reported AIDS cases (CDC 1998). Perhaps more striking is that in 1998, for women between the ages of twenty-five and forty-four, HIV/AIDS was the tenth leading cause of death among white women, the fourth leading cause of death among Latinas, and the third leading cause of death among African-American women (Kaiser Foundation 2001). Given that women of color are disproportionately represented among women with HIV/ AIDS, ideally blacks and Latinas would be overrepresented in this sample, but the selection processes and available resources did not allow for such discriminate recruitment. Therefore, any findings regarding women of color, specifically Latina women, are offered with caution. Research has found significant racial differences regarding social support, psychological well-being, formal service use, drug use, unmet need, negotiation of safe sex, and feelings about motherhood (e.g., El-Bassel and Schilling 1994; Levine 1990; Linn et al. 1995; Smith and Rapkin 1995; Wight, LeBlanc, and Aneshensel 1995). Given women's differential social place (including histories of discrimination and stigma) and conceptions of HIV/AIDS, it is likely that minority women think about and experience HIV infection in ways dissimilar to other respondents. Last, although it would be ideal to have respondents who represent different stages of the HIV/AIDS illness trajectory, the vast majority of the women in this sample did not suffer from opportunistic infections accompanying the virus or have full-blown AIDS. Further, although many did experience, at one time or another, common symptoms of HIV (e.g., recurrent vaginal yeast infection and fatigue) as well as other health problems which may or may not be HIV related, all reported good functional health. That is, very few of the women in this study were unable to independently tend to daily activities. Women's health, or the severity of their condition, may affect their perceptions of HIV infection and the distress caused by illness, which in turn can influence women's coping strategies. Moreover, in analyzing the impact of situations such as caregiving arrangements, functional health clearly impacts women's experiences. Relatively "well" women cannot speak directly to this issue, but can only speculate as to how their informal networks will respond when they are in need.

In-depth, semistructured interviews with respondents lasted anywhere from forty-five minutes to two hours; most lasted for an hour and a half. Interviews were transcribed verbatim and coded to organize emergent themes. To the extent possible, given the lengthy transcription process, transcripts were read and reread as they were transcribed. Timely coding of transcribed data allowed adequate familiarization with respondents and promoted interview guide reevaluation. Transcripts were initially coded for conceptual categories. Focused coding was then used to hone themes and develop analytic categories (Charmaz 1983a).

In the chapters that follow women's stories are presented and analyzed, particularly women's accounts of the disruptions caused by HIV/AIDS. The women's narratives express a wealth of suffering and healing, of disenfranchisement and empowerment. In fact, the extent to which these women articulated their defeats and triumphs was striking.

Feminist research methodology stresses the importance of the process of data collection, particularly the researcher's role in that process (Maynard and Purvis 1994; Oakley 1981; Reinharz 1992). Thus, at every stage of this research—from the original formulation of interview questions to the presentation of women's stories—a conscious attempt was made to present the women as experts on their experiences. In presenting and analyzing women's narratives, a concerted effort is also made to represent women's voices in a way that is true to their stories. Therefore, the excerpts throughout this book are presented verbatim and have not been corrected for grammatical errors. Instances in which words are interjected for clarity are identifiable and minimal so as not to detract from respondents' narratives.

Given the sensitive nature of the questions (e.g., sexual relations and illicit drug use), great pains were taken to assure women that the information they provided was completely confidential and would not interfere with the receipt of medical/social services. In addition, it was reiterated to respondents that they did not have to answer any question(s) that made them feel uncomfortable. Despite reservations, however, the women interviewed were incredibly open and freely offered many intimate details. Their candidness notwithstanding, as incomplete and reconstructed accounts their narratives do not perfectly reflect their actual experiences. As reproduced accounts, however, respondents strive to relay the "facts" of their stories as best they can. As women tell their life stories they strive to achieve coherence and continuity of self (Mishler 1992). That is, by recounting and pondering both the mundane and critical moments in their lives, they are better able to make sense of their lives and assert their identities. As Rosenwald and Ochberg (1992:5) note,

> The logic with which one event leads into another is not simply "out there," waiting to be recognized by any disinterested observer. Instead, coherence derives from the tacit assumptions of

plausibility that shape the way each story maker weaves the fragmentary episodes of experience into a history.

The interviewer also shapes women's narratives—from the topics chosen and followed up to the presentation of interview excerpts, this researcher actively participated in the reconstruction of each respondent's narrative (Mishler 1992).

OVERVIEW OF THIS BOOK

This chapter outlines the key issues and concepts explored throughout this book, including a discussion of the theoretical framework used to analyze the narrative data.

To elucidate women's illness experiences over time, Chapter 2 offers an analysis of how women initially experienced HIV infection. More specifically, Chapter 2 analyzes women's responses to their diagnosis, the meanings they attach to HIV/AIDS, and how learning of their HIV infection has affected their sense of self.

Health and illness are situated and managed in an individual's daily life. To more fully understand women's experiences with HIV infection we must gain a better understanding of how, and to what extent, they restructure their everyday lives to manage and cope with their illness, as well as the obstacles to such reorganization. Chapter 3 then looks at the daily obstacles or issues facing women with HIV infection and how their experiences compare to those of others with chronic illness.

Chapter 4 describes women's styles of legitimation or repair work, including going public with their illness, joining support groups, strengthening or establishing religious/spiritual ties, and using avoidance/denial modes. In analyzing women's responses, the benefits and potential shortcomings of these coping strategies are shown, and how this information is critical to serving women with HIV/AIDS is discussed.

Given the prevalence of informal caregiving among the chronically ill, it is important to establish the role of women's informal networks. Disclosure may be a key mechanism in marshaling social support. On the other hand, the decision of whether to tell loved ones and friends of the diagnosis is often a key problem and source of strain.

Chapter 5 examines the impact of significant others and social support networks in women's experiences with HIV/AIDS.

Relatively little is known about the role of caring in HIV-positive women's lives. Literature is quick to note how women's multiple caring roles, especially mothering roles, are compromised by illness. We are thus left with an image of women who are ill, lack social and material resources, and yet must struggle to care for their children and, often, other adults. Much less is known, however, about how women positively perceive their role as caregivers and how performing their caring responsibilities may mediate disruption and foster repair. The role of caregiving for children and other adults in women's experiences with HIV infection is explored in Chapter 6.

Before concluding, Chapter 7 examines the place of HIV/AIDS in women's biographies relative to other assaults on the self. When asked to compare HIV infection to other disruptions, many women reconstruct the initial meanings they attached to the virus and conclude that the illness is not the most disruptive life event they have experienced. Also disentangled are the factors that differentiate those for whom HIV was the most disruptive life occurrence from those for whom it was not. In addition, policy implications for the treatment of women with HIV/AIDS are outlined.

Chapter 8 summarizes the book's main themes and elaborates on women's coping and the potential problems that some women may experience as a result of their coping strategies. The role of women's informal and formal networks is highlighted in their experiences with HIV/AIDS. This chapter also discusses broader issues relating to empowerment and social change as well as the theoretical implications of this research.

Chapter 2

"Feeling Like Nothing": Receiving an HIV Diagnosis and Initial Disruption

Initially labeled Gay-Related Immune Deficiency (GRID), HIV/ AIDS has retained much of its deviant status. The identification of risk groups, rather than risk factors, has helped maintain the stigma of the disease (Weitz 1991) and has homogenized diverse groups (Schiller, Crystal, and Lewellen 1996). Subsequently, society seems to have adopted the attitude that intravenous drug users, the poor, and/or members of minority groups are the ones who contract—and deserve to contract—the virus while society's "desirables" do not. Many of the women in this study were aware of these social constructions even if they weren't exactly sure how to frame them. For these women, such social constructions went beyond academic discourse and were part of their lived experiences and identities.

BIOGRAPHICAL DISRUPTION AMONG WOMEN WITH HIV/AIDS

When recounting their experiences, these women explained how HIV has directly or indirectly affected most aspects of their lives and how it has shaped their identities. As noted in previous examples, HIV infection has had positive as well as negative ramifications. This chapter concentrates on the latter, as it was usually much later that these women discovered the ways in which HIV reinforced positive aspects of their identities. Specifically explored are women's reactions to the diagnosis and how finding out they have HIV infection affected their senses of self.

Being diagnosed with HIV infection was a traumatic event for most of the women in this sample. Reflecting nationwide trends, most are in high-risk behavior categories, i.e., they have histories of intravenous drug use and/or promiscuous sex. Many have struggled to clean up their act by enrolling in drug treatment programs to regain custody of their children and to maintain more healthy intimate relationships. Many aspire to lead normal lives. For these women, HIV posed a serious threat to the laborious work they had done to feel normal and gain positive senses of self. Initially, therefore, they could not conceive of a place for HIV in their biographies.

Clearly, one's interpretation of HIV infection affects whether it is considered to have a disruptive or reinforcing effect on one's biography. Although these women experienced various and multiple reactions to the knowledge of their diagnosis, the most typical reaction was hopelessness. Hopelessness, depression, and suicidal ideation are common reactions to being diagnosed with HIV infection (Jenkins and Coons 1996; Moneyham et al. 2000). Indeed, relative to non-HIV-infected individuals, people with HIV demonstrate a greater tendency toward suicidal thoughts and may be at greater risk for attempted suicide (Belkin et al. 1992). HIV-positive people with drug addictions appear to be at particular risk for suicide, as the multiple stressors they face, including poor physical and mental health and social isolation, are predisposing factors (Klee 1995). In their narratives, the women in the sample highlight the barriers that HIV infection poses to future goals and the often fatal nature of HIV/AIDS. Other common reactions include disbelief, social isolation, blame, and concern for significant others.

HOPELESSNESS

Upon diagnosis, many women (49 percent, $n = 18$) lost their will to go on. Five contemplated killing themselves, and two attempted suicide. Those with drug-use histories were more likely to report that they responded to their diagnosis with hopelessness compared to women without drug-use histories (81 percent and 19 percent, respectively). Indeed, many women expressed that as recovering drug addicts they were finally coming to a place in their lives where they were feeling good about themselves and that HIV jeopardized their progress. Even women who were still using drugs viewed themselves as close to getting clean prior to diagnosis; they may not have kicked their habits, but they were on the way. In light of their diagnoses, these women's perceptions of their progress may in part represent self-delusion. Regardless of how close they truly were to getting clean, they acknowledged their drug use as a problem that paled in comparison to receiving "a death sentence."

White women were more likely than women of color to have experienced hopelessness (75 percent and 25 percent, respectively). Although the women in this sample are fairly similar in terms of drug-use history and socioeconomic status, this finding may reflect the additional burdens faced by women of color by virtue of their race. Feeling desperate, a few women, such as Denise in Chapter 1, initially returned to drugs to deal with their diagnosis. Alcohol and drug binges or relapses are typical responses to being diagnosed with HIV infection (Jenkins and Coons 1996). A few respondents noted that the desperation produced by the knowledge that one has a life-threatening sexually transmitted disease interrupted their drug recovery progress. These women echoed Adele's sentiment: "Shit, I might as well go out and do drugs again."

Laurie experimented with intravenous drugs but says her cocaine addiction was the real problem. She had been clean for three years and had been living with HIV infection for about six years at the time of this study. Recounting what was going on in her life prior to being diagnosed, Laurie recalled that she was about to be married, and that she and her fiancé were tested as part of the routine prenuptial preparations. Her test results did not change her marriage plans, but her life changed forever. Feeling as though her life was over, Laurie turned to drugs and eventually lost custody of her children. In her words:

> He came back negative, I came back positive. I called off the wedding, but we ended up getting married, and it was an abusive relationship—it was a drug-filled relationship. I think part of it too was my HIV. I had found out I was HIV positive: I had no life; I didn't want to live. What good was I gonna be? I was gonna die anyway. So that's why I went to the drugs. I lost my kids, you know what I mean?

Being often solely responsible for the care of dependent children is a frightening ordeal for women with HIV/AIDS. Indeed, mothers of young children were especially likely to respond to their diagnosis with despair (i.e., of those responding with hopelessness, 76 percent were mothers, whereas 25 percent did not have any children). For women in this study with children, HIV infection signified not only premature death but also leaving their children motherless. Jessica, for example, a recovering addict and noncustodial mother of two, planned to regain custody of her children when she "got [her] act together." When she was given her diagnosis, she recalled immediately thinking about what her death would mean for her children:

> [I cried] "No, my God, my babies!" Matter of fact, I had brought my daughter to the doctor's with me at the time; she was about two years old. She was with me and I just was like, "Oh my God, my children are not gonna have a mother."

Carmen, one of the few Latina respondents, lives with her three children who range in age from three to eleven. Carmen is a lively young woman who has struggled to care for her children as a single parent while simultaneously battling her cocaine addiction. Describing herself as a former "drug addict and prostitute" who was "always in the streets," she also experienced great despair and suicidal thoughts: "I wanted to die, I wanted to die. I said, 'My life is over.' I attempted suicide two or three days after. I said, 'That's it, I don't have nothin' to live for.'"

Carolyn, forty-seven years old, found out she had HIV four years prior to the study. She is divorced and has two adult children. She did not have a drug-use history or many sexual partners, but she decided it was wise to be tested when she learned that her ex-boyfriend had tested positive. Upon receiving her diagnosis, Carolyn immediately associated HIV with AIDS, and hence death:

> Total shock, you just go numb. It must be the adrenaline. It's like a hot flowing sensation all through your body—it's just like a hot fluid goes through [you] . . . I was in shock. . . . Nothing meant anything to me. Of course, immediately you've got a death sentence; that's just what you stand there thinking.

Suspecting one may be positive does not alleviate feelings of despair. Kelly is a very lonely woman who lives by herself in a mobile home and very rarely interacts with others. She socializes mostly with her birds and dogs, treating them with great affection, as parents treat their children. At age forty-eight, Kelly has been divorced for nineteen years and has not been involved in any close relationships since. She has a twenty-nine-year-old son, who was raised primarily by his father and rarely initiates contact with his mother. In addition to HIV, Kelly has struggled with bulimia, clinical depression, and heroin addiction. Kelly had been clean for three years and had been living with HIV for about five years at the time of this study. She received her diagnosis when she was finally making clinical progress with her eating disorder and drug addiction, a diagnosis that threatened all of her hard work:

> It was so hard. I always kept thinkin' that it's almost like God gave me [a second chance]. I started feeling better for the first time. I was doin' really good, and it was like, "Wow, why? Why when I'm doin' good and for the first time?" I don't feel all screwed up, I'm not on a whole bunch of medication, and I find out that my life's gonna be short. And at that time I thought it would be shortened more than what I think now. . . . I figured maybe five or six years that I would have. But now I just don't wanna deal with people, [including] men. It's gettin' me more to be by myself, I think.

Despite her suspicions that she had HIV, the news was a blow, particularly since Kelly had no supportive people in her life to comfort her: "I had nobody to come home and talk to about it, I have been very much alone." Indeed, women in other studies have noted the need for greater support, particularly at the time of diagnosis (Heath and Rodway 1999).

Prior to her diagnosis, Nancy also suspected she might be infected with HIV. Nancy suffers multiple health problems, the most serious of which is emphysema. Nancy has had a long history of drug use and prostitution. She was not sure how she contracted HIV, but knew she would test positive:

> I've been in every category to get it: I've had blood transfusions. I've been a prostitute. When I had a [drug] habit . . . we all shared works, you know, 'cause there were tons of us. . . . So I've been in every [transmission] category, from the blood to the streets to sharing the works. . . . I just knew I was gonna come back positive. I knew because all the people I got high

with and everything and it's so widespread out there. It was inevitable, it had to be.

Reflecting on whether finding out she had HIV affected how she viewed herself, Nancy emphasized the fatal nature of HIV/AIDS and how ignorance heightens fear:

> Oh yeah, of course it does. They didn't have all the strides, you know, five years ago that they do now. So then that's what I felt like, I was gettin' clean you know? I didn't want to get clean just to turn around and die, you know? And that was like what I felt. And it was like learnin' it because you don't really know a lot until there's a reason to learn it, and so then I had to learn a lot more.

When asked if having HIV has affected her self-esteem or has made her feel like less of a good person, Nancy revealed that she is still grappling with the effects of the virus on her sense of self, specifically in terms of forming intimate relationships: "Yeah, I still have a hard time with that . . . because I've had a couple of bad experiences."

DISBELIEF

Other respondents (46 percent, $n = 17$) concentrated less on the consequences of HIV/AIDS and more on the inconceivability of contracting the virus. This response was especially common for women who contracted the virus via heterosexual sex as opposed to intravenous drug use (63 percent and 35 percent, respectively). Respondents in low-risk categories often questioned their diagnosis, which was not surprising. "How did I contract the virus?" many thought. "After all, I didn't shoot up; I wasn't promiscuous."

When asked to describe her reaction, for example, Alicia noted her low-risk lifestyle, and that as a single parent she was doing what she considered socially desirable and admirable—she was struggling to take care of her family without government assistance:

> I might have done a line here, or bag there . . . I was never a pig, or a whore, quote, unquote. When I first found out, I said, "Damn, man, why me? I ain't never did this, I never did that, I was never bad." I was a good mother, took care of my kid, you know, worked, wasn't on welfare.

Rachel also explained that given her sexual past and drug-use history she was at low risk for contracting the virus. Rachel is a thirty-two-year-old woman of Cuban ancestry who has been living with HIV infection for seven years. The abusive man who infected her had AIDS but never told her and in fact tried to make *her* feel responsible for infecting *him*. Rachel explained:

> He was very abusive. . . . By the time I found out he had this dark side, it was too late. I really couldn't get out, you know? . . . He had full-blown AIDS, I didn't even know. He'd get sick and say, "Oh, that's pneumonia." He'd go in the hospital and I didn't know, so I guess I wasn't as informed as I thought. . . . He would say things like, "Oh, would you be willing to die with me, the man you love?" You know, that kind of crap. And he would say, "There's been talk around town that you have AIDS and you were trying to give me AIDS." I was so confused, he was using this psychology on me and it really worked. So he'd turn around and make me think that I had it, and then I was like, "Yeah, but if I had it, why are you so sick?" "No, that's impossible," he says. "No, you bitch." And he'd beat me.

When he became seriously ill, Rachel decided she had better be tested. She was confident though that her low-risk lifestyle coupled with her knowledge of HIV transmission protected her against HIV/AIDS:

> I didn't have a lot of sexual partners. . . . I thought you'd have to have [sex] a lot of times to get it. . . . I did some drugs, I did some cocaine and I figured if I don't shoot up I can't get it either, you know, I was under that impression. . . . And I would read a lot about HIV, which is interesting. I would read a lot about it, and I would try to get as informed as I could, so I thought, "Okay, I'm not in the high-risk group, so there's no way."

Ten years prior to being diagnosed with HIV infection, Heather was "just more or less enjoying life." Having never used drugs, Heather was somewhat taken aback when her boyfriend of three months suggested they both be tested before they begin a sexual relationship. Admiring her new beau's consciousness about HIV/AIDS and feeling confident that she would test negative, she agreed to be tested. He tested negative, and she was shocked that she did not:

I guess the biggest feeling was one of disbelief. And I remember saying, "Could you be wrong?" She told me that the chance of her being wrong was probably something less than one percent. But I did go on to have another test and of course it came back positive, so then I was one hundred percent positive. . . . It was a death sentence she was giving me because back in 1988 they certainly didn't have anything near what they have today. And I just couldn't believe it. I didn't have a clue, I didn't even think there was a possibility.

Some women with high-risk histories also had a difficult time believing they could be HIV positive, highlighting many women's ignorance of virus transmission prior to their diagnosis. Those who engaged in high-risk behaviors often blurred the connection between their actions and transmission of HIV/AIDS. Becky, as with Denise and Laurie, did not think her drug use would have such devastating effects. When these women thought of risky behavior, they thought primarily of indiscriminate sexual relations. In addition, Becky distinguished functional drug users from nonfunctional ones—the former are able to lead productive lives and are thus safer than those addicts who lacked the will or resources to protect themselves. Thinking she was safe from the threat of HIV/AIDS, it was difficult for her to accept her diagnosis:

When two women came back in the room to tell me the results I knew something was up, and I was like, "No!" I'm very ignorant to a lot of things, and I thought well, I'm a clean person, you know, I keep my body clean. I've got good hygiene and always have, even on the drugs. 'Cause there's different degrees to go with our addiction, and at that point I've always had my own place, always had some money coming in. Sometimes not from straight-up resources, but I wasn't whoring or prostituting or anything like that, you know? Anyway, I went and had another [test] and it was also [positive]. . . . I went through some denial for a while thinking maybe they're wrong, you know?

Similarly, Laurie also recalled the shock and disbelief she experienced when receiving her test results. She suspected she may have a sexually transmitted disease, but not HIV/AIDS. She described her reaction:

I literally collapsed on the floor, my legs gave out and every-thing. Broke down uncontrollably, couldn't speak, couldn't breathe, nothing . . . I was in total shock, total shock. You know, it's like, "Why me?" I mean, up until that point I was like every-body else, you know, "Oh, only prostitutes get it, or gay people, or drug users." I'm none of that, so why should it happen to me? Now what's gonna happen? I felt like garbage. That's why I called off my wedding and everything. I said, "You deserve something better than this" and [he] was like, "No, I want you." It was total devastation.

Interestingly, despite her experimentation with intravenous drugs, Laurie did not consider herself at risk of contracting HIV. Having not been a "hard-core" addict, she interpreted her behavior as less harm-ful than what she considered typical drug users.

As with Laurie, Julia experienced disbelief and a sense of un-desirability. Julia, at the time of this study, had been living with AIDS for six-and-a-half years. She contracted the virus from her husband from whom she was divorced but was planning to remarry. Greg was an intravenous drug user and her sole sexual partner. When he found out he was HIV positive he urged Julia to be tested, assuring her that she would "be okay" because she has "never done anything wrong in [her] life; God wouldn't do that to [her]." Although she was aware of Greg's drug use, Julia explained that AIDS never crossed her mind:

AIDS was not as [publicized], it was still at that time some-thing you read in the back pages of the newspaper. It was just not a very prominent thing, it was still a gay man's disease. Well, it was filtering into the drug population, but mainstream America still wasn't being concerned with it. And even though I was aware of his drug history, that never entered my mind. I was brought up in the culture, like the late 1960s, early 1970s, like just don't get pregnant. It wasn't the disease thing; it was just don't get pregnant. I'm protecting myself from getting pregnant, so I'm okay. . . . It just didn't occur to me. It didn't occur to him either. It just did not.

Julia recounted her experience of receiving and denying her diagno-sis:

And I went in there and this lady, she hands you this eight and a half by eleven piece of white paper. [It] just slides across the desk in front of you with a number in the corner and all it says in the middle is "HIV positive." And I just looked at it and slid it back at her and said, "That's not mine." She says, "Yes, Julia, this is yours." And she slides it back at me. I said, "No, it's not. I want to see my paper. That's not my paper."

Julia checked the numbers on her card and despite the fact that they matched those on her test results, she again slid the paper back, insisting it was not her test: "I want to see *my* paper. I was so insistent. I want to see one that said HIV negative, basically was what I was telling her." Upon returning home, Julia broke down. She described that period as one of "total aloneness." Feeling overwhelmed and bewildered, she questioned her desirability. She felt trapped and could not imagine "who would ever talk to [her], who would want to be with [her]."

Repeated testing was common among women who were in disbelief. After subsequent test results confirmed their seropositivity, they were forced to face the fact of HIV infection. The threat of an untimely death and the very real fear that their children would lose their mother prematurely were extremely painful issues. In fact, some women denied their illness rather than face these eventualities.

Short-term users, as did "functional" users, also experienced disbelief. Michelle was introduced to heroin when she was eighteen years old. Two years later she found out she was HIV positive. She was given her test results in jail, secluded from the support of others. She explained:

I was just devastated, I couldn't believe it. . . . It was done in prison so it's not that comforting. I mean, they just had somebody talk to me. They said, "What do you think it is?" And I said, "I don't know." I said it really nonchalant like, "Yeah, I probably do," but I really didn't think I did. And when she said it, "It is positive," I just broke down. And there was a girl that I was really close to in there, and I was like, "Can you please get her?" And they couldn't find her, and I was already in a different section of the jail by then . . . and I was just like, "Please get her for me." And they couldn't find her and I just remember goin' back and I just didn't talk to anybody. . . . I kinda just denied it. I couldn't believe it.

Michelle's shock regarding her diagnosis stems from the fact that she was using drugs for a relatively short period:

> I was only usin' for a short period of time. I was like "Why me? I can't believe this; there's people I know that have been shootin' dope for twenty years!" You know what I mean? And here I was, I just went down so fast, I just lost everything so fast. When people have taken years and years to get to where I was. I just couldn't believe what was happenin', how quickly it was happenin' to me . . . and I used to be mad as hell 'cause I used to be like here I am, I went out there for a year and a half and I've already been to jail and I've lived on the streets and I've sold everything, I sold myself. And now I got this on top of it. . . . I feel like, why me? I really did question. But then people say, "Why not you?" You know?

Others concisely described their reactions of disbelief as being "freaked" by their test results. Indeed, "freaked" was a common adjective used by women to express the shock they experienced. As one woman put it, "I fuckin' freaked. I fuckin' freaked out, I didn't wanna hear nothin' else at all. . . . That fuckin' freaked me right out!"

SOCIAL WITHDRAWAL

HIV infection also diminished women's self-esteem and, for some, led to greater social isolation. Upon receiving their diagnosis, several women in this sample (16 percent, $n = 6$) indicated a reluctance to be socially active. Women who did not have intravenous drug-use histories were more likely to report social withdrawal as a reaction to their diagnosis (72 percent versus 33 percent of IV drug users). Women without drug-use histories have likely not had to deal with anything as stigmatizing as HIV/AIDS and, thus, have not felt the need to distance themselves from other people. Fear of rejection, abandonment, and discrimination were among the primary factors contributing to their social withdrawal. For women who did not know of anyone close to them with HIV, socializing was less appealing. For example, Thalia recalled: "When I first found out, I felt very dirty, very disgusting. Oh, God, it was sick! . . . I know nobody. It's like you feel like you're the only person on the planet. I feel like I'm the only person."

Similarly, Valerie said: "I know one thing: [HIV] makes you feel like nothing, you know what I'm saying?"

As with Valerie, Rachel felt worthless when she was diagnosed with HIV infection. Rachel is a vivacious young woman whose main hobby is reading. She spoke very quickly during the interview and thoughtfully demonstrated her interest and knowledge regarding HIV/AIDS and related issues. Speaking with Rachel, it is hard to imagine her being unable to interact with confidence. As she explained, however, there was a time when she did not feel comfortable talking to others much less coming into physical contact with them. In fact, simply speaking about her experiences would have been extremely difficult earlier in her disease process:

> At first you feel dirty. You know, I shouldn't even be in a room with you. I mean, I couldn't talk to you a few years ago, no way! Why would you want to be in here with me for? What are you, crazy?

These feelings and fears obviously had an impact on the women's social and familial relationships. As an egregious example, Rachel explained how her feelings of inadequacy and fear affected her relationship with her own child. Sadly, she recalled being afraid to show affection to her six-year-old daughter for fear of infecting her:

> Even though I knew you can't get it this way—and yet when I found out I had it, it was like, don't touch me, you'll get it. And I was so irrational, illogical. . . . I was afraid to hug my daughter. I was afraid that she would get it. . . . I couldn't hold her and she'd want to hold me and I would give her a light hug. But inside I just wanted to squeeze her. I mean, that's my baby.

However irrational, it took about a year for Rachel to overcome the fear of infecting her daughter, but occasionally these fears still creep in.

Part of the impact of HIV infection on the women's identities was how the virus ate away at their already tenuous self-assurance. As Kristen said:

> I don't feel as confident about myself as I used to and I'm shier. I always had a problem being shy and I think it's just made things more profound in that area. And I'm afraid of rejection as well, very much so, which is part of a lack of confidence.

Similarly, Stephanie described how she keeps to herself for fear of stigma and discrimination:

> I fear [that] if people find out they'll avoid me or possibly even discriminate [against me] in some way. . . . I understand. I don't necessarily blame them, I think maybe they're a little ignorant. But if they're afraid, that's one thing, as long as they don't do anything to try to hurt me, but that's also possible. . . . I just heard really bad stories in my [support] groups and I'm just going, "You've got to be kidding." So I don't want to expose myself to that. I don't see any reason to.

In addition to fearing negative reactions from others, some women figured it would be easier on them to not form relationships that HIV would destroy. For example, in the beginning Becky could not deal with being an HIV-infected woman. She did not think she was going to live much longer, so why bother to maintain or form relationships? Thinking in this fashion, she curtailed her social activities and became socially isolated. In her words: "I was very withdrawn and ashamed and stuff. I still can't believe it, you know. It's just like a dream. . . . I went through so much of the shame and everything . . . there was times when I was gonna be around for maybe another six months to a year, and I was just totally devastated."

PLACING BLAME

Although most women did not dwell on the origin of their infection or seek to place blame on themselves or others (mortal or divine), a few women (19 percent, $n = 7$) did express anger and blame toward those whom they believed infected them. The women in this study who had not used intravenous drugs were more likely to blame others for their infection than women with intravenous drug-use histories (71 percent and 29 percent, respectively). Women without drug-use histories generally do not feel as though they have engaged in high-risk behaviors, despite their sexual histories. Further, women who have had many sexual partners may not view their promiscuity to be as aberrant as needle sharing.

Debra, for example, blamed her ex-boyfriend for taking her off guard and sticking her with a contaminated needle. Debra told the story in this way:

> The morning [my son] was born . . . he was there very early Saturday morning with a syringe. There was a tinge of blood in it. And I was really groggy, and he said, "You deserve this. You look horrible, you've been through a lot." Boom, the next thing I know it was in my arm, and it was over. By the time I was aware I was already feeling the effects. I later found out that that was planned. . . . I feel like he signed my death warrant.

As this analysis shows, not all women with "someone to blame" condemned others. For example, Denise explained that she contracted the virus as a result of being raped, but, unlike Debra, she did not emphasize her assailant's part. Regardless of whether these atrocities led to their contracting HIV, they choose to interpret their situation and base the meaning of HIV/AIDS on these instances. Although their primary reactions to their diagnoses differed, their construction of how they contracted HIV illustrates how individuals may identify an incident that allegorically signifies their illness.

The pervasive negative images surrounding HIV/AIDS may well lead to internalized stigma, fostering feelings of self-condemnation and guilt (Lawless, Kippax, and Crawford 1996). By taking responsibility for their actions, few women blamed themselves for contracting HIV. Heather, however, did blame herself because after her first marriage she had been intimate with a few men and felt that in engaging in sexual relations she had strayed from her "original morals and standards":

> I couldn't blame anybody else. Whoever infected me, I don't know if they even knew they were infected so I can't say, "Well, he did this to me on purpose." Yeah, I did blame myself. I think if I were more responsible . . . I never took IV drugs and I never had a blood transfusion, but during those years from the time I was divorced till the time I remarried, I think it was in the early 1980s—1981, 1982—during those three years I sort of lost touch with my morals. And, you know, I just thought 'cause I was brought [up] as [a] strict Catholic, and having been brought up that way, I was a virgin when I was married. . . . After I got divorced I thought, now what do you do? Like what's the rule

now? You kind of live by rules all your life. You can't go back, but I just wish I had sought out some advice from somebody that I could trust. Not that I became promiscuous right then and there after I got divorced, but by the time, like almost a decade later like in the early 1980s, I had reached a point where I thought "well, it's okay." And there were at least—it wasn't any more than ten. But it only takes one time.

Heather noted that when the reality of her situation set in and her guilt alleviated, she was still left to deal with feelings of worthlessness: "When I first found out I felt like I was damaged goods. Like if I was in a market, I'd be on sale. Just get it out of the store!"

Other women were angry with God because He failed to protect them despite their faith and/or low-risk behavior. Lisa lost her youngest daughter, Marisa, to AIDS. She never used drugs and contracted the virus from her ex-husband who was an IV drug user. She described her reaction to her diagnosis:

I was so angry with God. I was brought up Catholic and the only thing I ever asked for whenever I either prayed or went to church, I just would say, "Keep my kids safe from harm and illness." That's all I ever asked for. I was so angry.

During her interview, Jocelyn expressed that she was very unhappy with the way [her] life was going. She felt that combined with HIV the trouble she was having raising her two adolescent daughters were part of a divine punishment for not practicing safe sex. However, it was at her lover's request that they stopped using condoms:

[In addition to] the virus and I'm havin' trouble with my kids . . . and I have bad luck every day. I think God's just punishing me . . . for what I did. . . . You know I was goin' with him for—well, we been goin' together for five years . . . but let me tell you this one, that five years we was usin' condoms, them whole five years, you understand me? And so that one day I didn't use one, okay. I swear on my mother's [soul] we was usin' condoms, and so two years later he just started sayin' he wasn't comfortable with them. You know, and he's fifty years old.

PUTTING ONESELF LAST

In line with traditional gender roles, some respondents (14 percent, $n = 5$) discussed the disruption caused by HIV in terms of its effect on their husbands or lovers. Women without intravenous drug-use histories were more likely to be concerned about the impact of HIV on their loved ones (60 percent versus 40 percent of women who used drugs). For some women, drug use had precluded active involvement in caring roles. In addition, active users may not have been in a state of mind to think about the welfare of others. As the nurturers and health care organizers for their families, women who put themselves last were not immediately concerned with the effect of the virus on their own health. Rather, they worried about how it would affect their loved ones. Unlike the women in previous examples, these respondents did not emphasize the fatal nature of the disease or loss of future aspirations. Instead, they highlighted the infectious nature of HIV.

Robyn had HIV infection for seven years at the time of the study, which she contracted from heterosexual sex. Despite her battle with alcoholism, Robyn always managed to perform her job as a nurse at an assisted-living center. She and her boyfriend were both tested— his test results came back negative, hers were positive. This did not anger her; rather, she was concerned with how *her* having HIV would impact *him*. She said, "I was just kind of more afraid of how it was gonna affect him and the relationship, more than the fact that I would die."

Initially, Adele did not think about what HIV infection meant for her life and health either. Rather, as with Robyn, she immediately worried about infecting her lover: "First thing I thought was I hope I didn't give it to my boyfriend. I mean that would be the ultimate . . . I could handle her telling me I had it, but I couldn't have handled it if he was positive, which he isn't, thank God." In fact, Adele described how for months she felt she was a danger to others: "I mean [me] havin' it is one thing. I don't wanna pass it to nobody, you know what I mean? And for awhile there, every time I would bleed I would feel like hey, I'm a walking killer here."

Women who put off dealing with their diagnosis, or downplayed its effects, were often occupying caregiving roles when they found out that they were HIV positive. A few respondents were caring for their HIV-infected husbands/lovers when they received their diagnosis. These women did not feel that they had much time to think about their own health; their everyday caring labor did not allow time for conscious integration of HIV infection into their biographies. Only in retrospect, since many are no longer primary caregivers, can they reflect on what HIV means to and for them. Hillary, for example, did not get her test results promptly because she was busy caring for her dying husband. She said:

> I'm so busy keeping him going, to fight for his life and not give up, that I didn't think about me. And those two weeks that I had to wait for the results, they went by pretty quickly. And the doctor never said anything, and one day it dawned on me, it's been over two weeks, so I asked.

Similarly, for the first year following her diagnosis Donna did not really acknowledge her illness because she was busy caring for others—working as a certified nursing assistant in a nearby nursing home and caring for the father of her children, who died of AIDS in 1995. As Donna explained:

> I was diagnosed [in] 1994. But it just didn't hit me right away what was goin' on and I tried to just keep on with my life— workin' and takin' care of him, and it got a little bit much so then I just said [to myself], forget the job, just totally take care of him. So then I had no income and he had no income and my daughter had little kids, so we all [had to] make it work. But it was really stressful, I lost so much weight. Didn't have much hair.

Sheila was also caring for her dying husband when she received her diagnosis. Sheila described her first marriage as a mistake; she was young and naive and "didn't know what love was." Pregnant with his child, Sheila saw marriage as the only option. She wanted to leave him early on, but her parents strongly discouraged her. After enduring years of abuse, she finally saved up enough money to "run away." In addition to being violent, Sheila's husband also concealed his drug-use history and the fact that he had AIDS. Sheila took care of him until his death despite that fact that he hurt her and, in her opinion, maliciously infected her.

As with Donna, Sheila too reported a delayed response to her test results:

> It's gonna sound strange, it might sound stupid, but I had no thoughts. It was like I didn't know what to think. . . . I didn't have any feelings about it. I really didn't know what it was, you know what I mean? So I was like, "Okay, fine." And [the doctor] said, "You're handling this pretty good." What am I supposed to say? What am I supposed to do? And I knew that my husband was dying. . . . I didn't have a car. I didn't even know how to drive, so I ended up catching the bus home. . . . I remember him telling me at that time what my count was. I remember saying, "Thank you very much."

These women were too preoccupied with their caring duties to devote time to their own health and illness. In fact, they were much more likely to delay even thinking about what HIV meant for them. As will be discussed in Chapter 6, these women had additional material (i.e., caregiving experiences) from which they could reconstruct their narratives.

ASSIGNING MEANING AND SENSE OF SELF

As the women in this study recount (and undoubtedly reconstruct) the disruption caused by HIV, they concentrate on the meaning of HIV couched in its consequences (Bury 1991), particularly mortality and maintaining and/or establishing intimate relationships. The majority of the women in this group clearly interpreted HIV as a serious, fatal disease. Most did not think they would live five, much less ten, years following their diagnosis. As one woman said, "I think that pretty much everybody goes through the same things. . . . A lot of things change because being HIV positive, or having cancer or whatever, makes you realize that you are mortal, and you are gonna die."

Given the terminal and stigmatized nature of HIV/AIDS, these women felt worthless, undesirable, and uneasy about their own as well as their children's health and futures. The ways in which these women experienced HIV in its early stages exemplify the reactions highlighted in the academic and popular literature on women and HIV/AIDS. As Kelly's response in an earlier example demonstrates, even those who suspected they were HIV positive, due to needle sharing and/or unprotected sex, experienced a ruptured sense of self. In fact, despite their hunches, when their premonitions were validated many of these women experienced shock and anger. It appears that their suspicions were of little help in preparing them for their results.

Internalizing the shame and stigma associated with HIV/AIDS, many women have come to view themselves in negative terms. These women saw themselves as "abnormal" and "dirty." As Sheila explained: "When I first found out I thought very low of myself, like I was dirt, I was filth. It was almost like back in the Bible how it says people had leprosy, like I would never be accepted." Similarly, Debra explained her sense of self as contagious:

> I sometimes see myself as one big germ. I used to have this dream . . . I'd wake up and go in the bathroom and open the medicine cabinet and there were these huge white bottles and they'd say, "Debra for AIDS." There were three rows of these bottles that say, "Debra for AIDS."

Valerie succinctly stated that HIV infection "makes you feel like nothing." Melissa said the virus makes her feel like "less of a good person."

Some of these women felt as if their positive status made it impossible for them to interact in normal social circles or form intimate relationships with normal lovers. Women who have internalized the social construction of the devalued person with HIV/AIDS did not feel worthy of interacting with noninfected people. As Michelle explained:

> I guess when I first found out I didn't feel worthy of having a decent boyfriend. I thought the only person I could get was maybe another junkie or somebody with the virus too. I didn't think I could get a normal person who didn't have a drug history and who didn't have the illness. I just went through a phase where I just was real disgusted with myself.

Indeed, the barriers imposed by HIV/AIDS in establishing intimate relationships was a central feature of these women's lived experiences. As will be discussed in Chapter 5, disclosing one's positive status to potential significant others is a major source of stress and a constant reminder of the disruptive nature of HIV infection.

A few women reported that their feelings of shame and stigma became acute when participating in social life. In the early years of living with HIV, for instance, Carolyn felt conspicuous, as if people knew that she was different—that she was infected:

> There were times when I'd be at work, or in a restaurant, or in a nightclub, and in the back of my mind I felt very different. Like if these people knew, I know I'm sticking out like a sore thumb.

Rose, who thought she was "on [her] way out" when she was diagnosed with HIV infection, also expressed that she felt conspicuously different or abnormal:

> I was very depressed in the beginning. I remember goin' to a baseball game and my son was playin' sports, and I remember sittin' there startin' to cry, lookin' around, thinkin', they're all right and I'm different. I had an awful feeling about it. . . . I mean that's how bad it was. I remember bein' in a grocery store thinkin' to myself, somebody's standing behind me writin' a check. Why am I [the way that] I am, and they're *regular?*. . . In the beginning I just felt like people could look at me and know . . . I just had a bad time.

These characterizations clearly illustrate the ramifications of life disruptions on women's senses of self. These women's narratives highlight the differences they perceive between normality and abnormality—the difference between being a regular person and being an unusual, if not deviant, person. It took Rose about a year to feel better about herself or at least to feel inconspicuous.

WOMEN AND DISRUPTION

As illustrated in the previous examples, the knowledge that one is HIV positive provoked women to recount and analyze their pasts, especially those whose histories included drug use and promiscuity. These women were similar to the gay men in Carricaburu and Pierret's (1995) sample in that both groups perceived HIV as disruptive, at least initially. Some of the women in this study had similarly organized their lives around hardships such as poverty, abuse, and drug addictions. Although organizing one's life around illness, especially a stigmatized illness, is very different than organizing one's life around hardships, especially those rooted in deviant behavior, both groups draw on past experiences to make sense of their current situation. Although many tried to put these times behind them, HIV infection made this impossible. Rather, HIV/AIDS brought these women's past behaviors and identities to the fore. They had to recollect their pasts to account for their present situation. Indeed, many of these women discussed HIV in terms of what they did or did not do to themselves in terms of risk of infection.

Although women recounted their histories, very few could salvage any empowering aspects from their pasts to help them incorporate HIV into their biographies with any ease. Prior to their infection, the gay men in Carricaburu and Pierret's (1995) sample had viewed their identity as homosexuals in positive terms. Further, they were able to draw strength and motivation from their struggles as an oppressed group. By virtue of their social place, women with HIV are indeed an oppressed group. Their sex, race, class, and drug addictions, however, have not been unifying characteristics. Most spoke of their personal, not their social, identities. For some women, HIV/AIDS led to the realization that they are part of a collective group, however disconnected, and that their actions can make a difference. As will be discussed in Chapter 4, HIV infection was the impetus for various types of group involvement for these women, most often via support groups for people with HIV/AIDS and participation in AIDS awareness/education efforts. For women with racial and class privilege, however, organizing with poor, minority women with HIV was not easy. Support groups were not that helpful to Stephanie, for example, because her problems and concerns seemed trivial compared to the disadvantaged women in her group.

Not surprising was it that women who were not drug users found it difficult to identify with those who were; women who were not poor found it difficult to identify with those living in poverty. Furthermore, women whose past identities were based on their drug addictions, or neglectful parenting did not want these aspects reinforced. These were aspects of self that they were working to reconstruct into more positive identities. Thus, for the women in this sample, HIV meant a reorganization and reconstruction of their biographies.

In this chapter, it has been shown how a group of women responded to the knowledge of their illness early on. Their feelings changed over the years as they have gone from diagnosis to living with HIV infection. As will be discussed in Chapter 3, over time the meanings attached to HIV and its effect on the women's sense of self have been reconstructed. Also, women based their self-concepts less on past identity and more on their present and anticipated future selves. These changes are undoubtedly grounded in their daily experiences. Thus, the following chapter explores the issues that they identify as most prominent in their daily lives.

Chapter 3

Living with HIV Infection:
The Impact of Illness on Everyday Life

Chronic disease diagnosis signifies the beginning of one's progression from healthy to ill. Illness alters one's participation in social life and relationships as well as one's sense of self. Chronically ill persons must adapt to, and manage, their illness trajectories—intermittent periods of sickness and wellness. The very knowledge that one has a fatal illness may interfere with daily living, even in advance of functional disabilities.

Gains and losses of self occur along the illness trajectory and are experienced in everyday life (Charmaz 1983b; 1991). Thus in analyzing the ways in which living with HIV has shaped women's identities, respondents' accounts of the effect of HIV on their daily lives were elicited. This chapter presents the primary obstacles women with HIV/AIDS face and compares their experiences with other populations, illustrating their unique illness experiences.

GENDER AND THE PSYCHOSOCIAL IMPACT
OF HIV INFECTION

The nature of the disease and its social construction produce similar challenges and issues for men and women, since it poses serious threats to physical and emotional well-being. However, as with most social phenomena, gender matters. Differences in social status, resources, roles, and responsibilities produce distinctive experiences and needs.

Similar to HIV-positive men, women with HIV/AIDS are faced with the physiological effects of the virus, functional decline, demanding treatment regimens, disclosure decisions, financial insecurity, and stigma and discrimination. Clearly, however, literature reflecting the experiences of middle- to upper-middle-class gay white men cannot be extrapolated to women with HIV infection. Women, particularly those with substance-abuse histories, face unique challenges that are not typically central concerns for their male counterparts, including poverty, caring for children and/or other adults, reproductive decisions, guardianship plans for dependent children, access to health care and social services, adequate housing, negotiating condom use, sexual undesirability, and abandonment (Carlson et al. 1997; Chung and Magraw 1992; Gillman and Newman 1996; Goggin et al. 2001; Henderson 1992; Semple et al. 1993; Weitz 1993). As noted in Chapter 1, race and class inequities exacerbate these problems (Fuller, Geis, and Rush 1988; Stuntzer-Gibson 1991; Ward 1993).

ADAPTIVE TASKS FOR WOMEN WITH HIV/AIDS

Respondents highlighted the social and physical aspects of living with HIV infection when talking about their daily lives. These concerns and problems reflect women with substance-abuse histories who are also single mothers, and who are uneducated and unskilled. As they talked about living with HIV, some highlighted concerns that were ever present but exacerbated by HIV. Others underscored the more physical and medical aspects of living with HIV/AIDS. Regardless of which concerns women emphasized, they explained how HIV impedes mundane activities. Further, despite their desire not to dwell on illness, several factors often resurface making this a difficult task. Fear of rejection and stigma, the difficulty involved in establishing intimate relationships, dealing with death and dying, and financial survival are the primary difficulties these women face.

Fear of Rejection and Stigma

As noted in Chapter 2, social isolation is a common occurrence among people with HIV/AIDS. Fear of rejection or abandonment often curtailed the women's social involvement. Concern with rejection and stigma appears to be more central for women who have histories of intravenous drug use (i.e., women who have used intravenous drugs were more likely to express a fear of rejection, 67 percent and 33 percent, respectively). This may be due to the fact that when these women were using drugs they had a circle of friends or "running buddies" (Friedman, Des Jarlais, and Sterk 1990) and thus felt accepted even if they were ostracized from other groups (e.g., their families). HIV-infected persons may not have a group of others in a similar situation to whom they feel connected. The presence of a significant other may also be a factor in women's assessments; that is, 56 percent of women who did not have a partner identified this concern versus 44 percent of women who had partners. Women who have not been rejected by their partners, those with whom they share most intimately, may worry less about rejection from other sources. Similarly, women who had been living with HIV infection for seven or more years at the time of this study were more likely to fear rejection than women diagnosed fewer than seven years prior to this study (56 percent and 44 percent, respectively). Women who had been living with HIV for a longer duration may have had more time to experience stigma, or to learn of others who had been rejected, and to view rejection as a more common response.

Carmen explained that her social circle shrank as a result of infection and that it is difficult getting close to people because she fears rejection. When asked about her friendships, she said:

> I don't let people get too close to me. I don't know what type of reaction [I would get] if they were to find out, so I prefer not to. Because I had one experience with a friend, me and her got real close, and then a year later I decided to tell her and I never seen her again.

In fact many of the women interviewed did not have very many friends before they became infected, and HIV seemed to exacerbate their reticence to become socially involved, especially with people without HIV/AIDS. Becky would like to form close friendships with such people, and possibly become romantically involved, but she is protecting herself emotionally by "playing it safe":

> I do get angry sometimes. I get fearful because I believe that I'm ready to date or have friends, [but] the way I see some people react—part of me is afraid for that hurt so I don't set myself up for it. Because I'm very safe right now, very safe in my emotional health. . . . My point is I get angry too, and I think, "Why does that have to get in my way?"

What emerges from these women's narratives is their sense of perceived difference. They have come to distinguish themselves from seronegative people and often feel unworthy to gain entry into their social world. Attempts to submerge their infected selves can be strenuous and at times fruitless and, as in Becky's case, extremely frustrating. For Kristen, the psychosocial effects of not fitting in are the most difficult part of living with HIV infection:

> And just gettin' a little depressed sometimes [because] I feel like I'm different from most people. And even if I go somewhere, to a party or something like that, and everybody's having a good time, I always feel alienated. And there may be other people there that may be HIV positive but that they don't even know. But I always just feel like that . . .

Anticipated rejection or perceived stigma is a powerful force that circumscribes women's social involvement. Enacted stigma, on the other hand, affirms women's fears and presents a very real barrier to participation in social life. For instance, since being diagnosed five years prior to this study, Kelly has dated a couple of men. Upon learning of her serostatus, however, both men broke off contact with her. Because of these negative experiences, Kelly has lost her will to be socially active:

> One night I remember we went out and we was talkin' and I said, "I got something to tell you. In my past life I kinda screwed up a little bit, and things happened, and I'm HIV positive." They both stopped calling me. So I guess I'm just too afraid to go through that, I don't wanna go through that. . . . At one time I was goin' to singles dances. . . I got the rejection because of my HIV and [now] I just don't go out.

A couple of women described instances of discrimination in employment, but most respondents described less blatant instances of rejection and discrimination. Not surprisingly, avoidance from family members and friends was the most painful type of rejection. Even those who seem supportive have their moments of fear and engage in hurtful actions. Michelle recalled an incident in which her father, with whom she had a close relationship growing up, tried to keep her away from his other children for fear of infection:

I can remember one Christmas I called up and I was like, "Do you want me to come by?" And he's like, "Yeah, all right." And he had called back and told me that he didn't think it was a good idea for me to come over because there was kids there. And I was like, "What?" And I didn't talk to him for a long time after that 'cause that really, really hurt me. You know, I can understand bein' scared, but this was a parent and he was just really, really ignorant.

Michelle did not talk to her father for over a year after that incident. She was most angered by the fact that her father apparently made no attempt to educate himself about HIV/AIDS, but rather relied on myths and stereotypes about transmission of the virus:

I know if I had a kid and my daughter told me that she had something, I would look it up. I would find information on it. I would know that you couldn't get it through casual hand-holding or touching. And for my father to say that to me really, really hurt me. 'Cause he didn't even have the time to go and check in about it, ask about it, know that I'm not gonna give it to his kids.

Although Michelle said that she is much more open about her serostatus than when she was diagnosed with the virus seven years prior, her experience with her father contributes to her reticence to "go public":

And now a lot of people know—a lot of my close friends know and my family knows. But I'm not like open to it where I go and talk to groups because I still know there's just so much discrimination. There's still so much stigma. Even though it's a lot better, it's still not the way it needs to be, you know what I mean? And I'm not one to deal with that kind of people. . . . There are still people that are real ignorant about it. They just don't wanna learn anything about it until they're gonna have to, when it's like their kid or their niece or nephew. And it's too bad, but that's pretty basically the reality of it.

To combat negative reactions and discrimination, Michelle wished that HIV/AIDS would be treated more like other chronic illnesses:

I really think there needs to be way more funding than there is
for research, because I think if they at least just find some medication that we can live with this like it's diabetes or something.
It would just be like herpes or something like that, where there is
no cure for herpes but we can live with it. You still gotta have
protected sex. I just wish it was more something like that, that
they would find some medication that you can just really live for
the rest of your life with it, just like another virus. . . . I just hope
that they do find something.

Intimate Relations

Closely related to fear of rejection is the effect of HIV/AIDS on
women's romantic lives and sexual identities. In her personal account
of her experiences with breast cancer, Dorothy Becvar (1996:84) elo-
quently states a sentiment expressed by several of the women in this
sample: "I want you to know that, for a woman, breast cancer constitutes a 'double whammy.' Not only does it confront me with my own
mortality, it also assaults my basic identity and integrity, often leaving me feeling somehow less than a woman." Illness is one factor that
may shatter relationships or discourage individuals from romantic involvement. Unlike women with other illnesses, women with HIV/
AIDS may feel obligated to tell their partners that they have a sexually transmitted, life-threatening illness. They also face the possibility of being discredited by men who deem them indecent or promiscuous based on their seropositive status. For women in this survey
who were actively seeking companionship and intimacy, HIV chal-
lenged the way they think about sexuality and behave sexually. These
women have suffered a "sexual death," wherein their identity as desirable, sexual beings was threatened or, at worst, destroyed (Ross
and Ryan 1995). Not surprisingly, all of the women in this study who
highlighted this problem were at the time not involved in an intimate
relationship. Women who did not have an intravenous drug-use history were also much more likely than women with drug-use histories
to discuss the difficulty of establishing romantic ties (80 percent and
20 percent, respectively). As two respondents noted, HIV/AIDS had
severely circumscribed the dating pool. For example, if seeking HIV-
positive men, these women may be more susceptible to meeting men
with drug-use histories. Women with drug-use histories themselves,
on the other hand, were accustomed to dating men with substance-

abuse problems. Women who had been living with HIV infection for seven years or more were also more likely than those with the virus for fewer than seven years to highlight this problem (60 percent and 40 percent, respectively). Similar to their fear of rejection, women living with HIV for longer periods of time may have been trying to establish intimate relationships for a longer period of time, and their failure to find a suitable mate has become a marked concern.

Overall, the women surveyed in this research were very open about how the virus affected their intimate relationships. Kristen was very candid in discussing the impact of HIV on her sex life. The virus has not yet negatively affected her functional health so she has not had to curtail most of her prized activities, including spending time with her nineteen-year-old son. There is, however, one thing she used to enjoy but feels that her seropositive status has taken away: "Having sex! Yeah, right, that would be the big one." As the women described the impact of HIV/AIDS on their romantic lives, they agreed that disclosure is the hardest part of establishing relationships. Trying to anticipate and prepare oneself for the reactions of potential partners produces extreme anxiety. The first rejection is diminishing and it dampens any desire to try again; in other words, there is reluctance to set oneself up for another potential rejection. When asked about her intimate relationships, Jennifer responded quickly, and noted that HIV has threatened her sexual identity: "My sex life is nonexistent. You wanna know how long it's been since I got laid? It's been, good God, almost two and a half years! It is hard, especially since I always thought of myself as a very passionate, sexual human being." At the age of forty-five Jennifer has found it difficult to establish intimate relationships with men, despite her strong desire to become involved. She too appears to have internalized stigmatized conceptions of people with HIV/AIDS: She noted that if the tables were reversed—if a potential love interest told her that he had HIV/AIDS—she might reject him:

> The big difference in my life has been relationships. Having HIV really has, well, you know what I mean. I haven't had many relationships. I don't seek out men that are not [HIV] positive. Although this could be looked at as a chronic condition, it's not the same as having diabetes. And frankly, I put myself in another person's place, and no matter how wonderful a person I might be, I think this is a lot to put somebody through. And

I guess it's a defense mechanism too, protecting myself from re-jection. I don't wanna go out with somebody and then have to say, "Look, I got AIDS."

Although Jennifer seeks to avoid rejection by dating only men who are HIV positive, she does not feel completely at ease seeking out men from this pool of eligibles:

Frankly, I wasn't [sexually active] for a very long time, until some friends urged me: "Well, there's guys out there who have this disease." I said, "Yeah, but they're all ex-drug addicts." I mean, these are not men that I would have gone out with before!

HIV/AIDS has placed such women as Jennifer in a new social world—a place populated by people with whom she may not have previously come into contact, much less contemplate romantic in-volvement. Therefore, she sees her relationships as abnormal in the sense that she does not truly expect to form a lasting union. When asked what the most difficult part of living with HIV infection is, she replied:

Not being able to have a normal relationship, 'cause I guess I al-ways thought that eventually I would marry again. I never thought that I might be growing old alone, and having this dis-ease [makes it] very possible, a great possibility.

Death and Dying

In addition to the social impact of HIV, the women in this study discussed the physical or health-related consequences of being in-fected. This concern was especially common among women who had been living with HIV infection for seven or more years (82 percent versus 18 percent of those diagnosed fewer than seven years prior). It is likely that as these women approach the period when people with HIV infection typically develop AIDS or become symptomatic, the fear of mortality will be brought to the forefront. Women who had in-travenous drug-use histories were also more likely to worry about death and dying than women who had not used intravenous drugs (63 percent and 37 percent, respectively). Although we may expect women with drug-use histories to be less concerned with their health, these respondents may be worried that HIV infection, coupled with the harmful effects of their drug use, will exacerbate their ill health. In addition, by abstaining from drugs these women began to view themselves as relatively healthy, and HIV/AIDS threatened their progress. More women without partners highlighted this concern than women involved in intimate relationships (64 percent and 36 percent, respectively). The fear of death may be abated for women who have the support and assurance of a significant other.

Most frequently, women's concerns centered around death and especially dying. Indeed, later stages of HIV infection, or full-blown AIDS, are characterized by opportunistic illnesses and diseases causing a variety of conditions, including hair loss, skin problems, wasting, lymphomas, severe musculoskeletal pain, blindness, and cognitive impairment (Folkman, Chesney, and Christopher-Richards 1994; Brown 1996). Many described a constant waxing and waning of the fear of death. As Karen put it, "I go through stages of when I'm having panic attacks, 'I'm gonna die, I'm gonna die!' It's in the middle of the night and I'm up." Similarly, Nancy said one of the most difficult parts of having HIV infection is "the fear that you're gonna die, 'cause you always have that fear." These women are not only fearful for themselves, but they also worry about losing friends to the disease—of dealing with "a lot of death now."

Asymptomatic women must deal with the constant threat of sickness, although they cannot be certain of when their health will take a turn for the worse. Adele described her concerns regarding death and dying as "waiting for AIDS":

> I'm seein' a counselor 'cause it's like you're waiting for the other shoe to drop, you know? Like I went to this education program about AIDS and the man said a lot of people, believe it or not, feel a great relief when they go from HIV to AIDS. Because all the time before that you're waitin' for it. You know it's gonna happen, but you don't know when.

Adele's situation most vividly illustrates the social death associated with HIV/AIDS (Ross and Ryan 1995). The uncertainty of the onset of AIDS, and hence death, was so anxiety provoking that she withdrew from any social participation. In fact, she did not leave her house for about five years after she was diagnosed with HIV infection.

Even women who tried to remain optimistic and not dwell on sickness and death feared disease progression. They know that their status could change at any time—that they could develop AIDS. Michelle, similar to Adele, feels that it may not be long before her luck runs out. For her, this is the most difficult part of living with the virus:

> Knowing that there's no cure. Seeing and hearing other people around you die. Hearing the horror stories of how people die with AIDS . . . I've had the virus for about seven years now and I haven't been sick. Well, yeah, that's a good thing, but the longer you have it, you know, I kinda feel like, you know, when? When is it gonna happen? So you get kinda nervous. And I guess it's the not knowing—not knowing how you're gonna die.

AIDS signifies unfulfilled dreams and goals. Nancy would very much like to get her adolescent children on the right track before she dies. By her own admission, she was not a very good mother when her children were growing up. Drug use and prostitution led to Nancy losing custody of her three preadolescent children. The children bounced from their grandmother's home to their aunt's and uncle's custody to foster home placement, and thus she has had sporadic contact with her children and limited involvement in their lives. In fact, she gave up her youngest son for adoption when he was six years old and has not had much contact with him since then. She worries most about her eighteen-year-old son who, like his parents, has problems with drugs and alcohol. Given the unstable environments in which her children were raised, Nancy hopes that before she dies she will get the opportunity to see them leading stable, productive lives:

> I wanna make sure I don't go until I have these kids' lives settled. And Kate's [living] with her boyfriend; she's not totally settled but somewhat. Bobby, that kid's off the freakin' wall. He's more like me and [my ex-husband] than the other two. Oh God, I hope they are situated then it's not my time to go 'cause I don't wanna go right after that, you know? But that's like one of my most important things, just makin' sure that they're all, like, all right with their lives, you know?

Lisa explained that she is not afraid of death. In fact, when her daughter died of AIDS she saw death as the only way to deal with her pain and attempted to commit suicide. Lisa focused on the uncertainty surrounding HIV/AIDS and the unrealized goals left in its wake. In discussing the hardest part of living with HIV, she said, "Not having a future or not knowing the future. Which I mean nobody does [know the future], but it's like I don't plan things too far ahead . . . I also like don't think, 'Oh yeah, I'll have a house someday 'cause I know [I won't],'you know?"

Indeed, the contemplation of long-term plans brings the fatal nature of HIV/AIDS to the forefront. Having wasted time because of drug use or other barriers to productivity, the women must now contend with HIV/AIDS as an obstacle. Being asymptomatic and functional is not necessarily a consolation. At age thirty-two, Rachel is a young woman with great ambition and diverse interests. Drugs, single motherhood, and financial problems have kept her from realizing her potential. She dreams of getting a college education and pursuing a career in social service. Although she may take steps to better herself, she fears that before long she will be too sick to pursue her goals:

> Not being able to plan for something. Wondering when I'm gonna be sick. Even though I should be enjoying this time and be grateful for it, I'm sure when I do get sick I'm gonna say, "Damn, I wasted all that time again!" . . . I was going to computer school, but I messed up there because that's when things started happening, and I would say, "Oh, let's do a little cocaine," you know? I wasted so many years. It's incredible when you find out you don't have that many years left. You say, "Damn, I wasted a lot of years!"

When asked if she and her present partner have discussed marriage, she reiterated that HIV precludes them from making long-term plans. "Getting married and thinking about the future and having children, I can't do any of that." Even when consciously trying to focus on other areas of their lives, respondents were not always able to disregard their HIV status. Good health and joyous occasions are often interrupted by thoughts of the inevitability of illness and death. As Michelle explained:

> Sometimes I think about [HIV/AIDS] when I don't want to, and that sucks. I'll be havin' like a really good time. I'll be on vacation, I'll be in Florida with my friends doin' somethin'. All of a

sudden I think about it. It gets me depressed, you know? Or somebody will be talkin' about years from now or when I'm forty, and I'm thinkin' to myself I might not make it. Then I start thinkin' I might not be here when I'm forty.

Perhaps more disconcerting than facing one's mortality is facing a painful death. As the women recounted the struggles associated with living with HIV infection, they highlighted their fear of physical and mental deterioration. Many echoed Kelly's sentiment: "I was afraid of the way I'd go, the pain and suffering and everything else that goes with it." Michelle also explained that she is frightened by the physical changes (e.g., wasting) and increased or total dependence on others:

> There's just so many things that I don't wanna go through. I don't wanna be losin' my mind and be seventy pounds and in diapers. I just can't. I would just say, "Please, just let me die before that." There's just no way I would wanna live like that, you know? And I wouldn't want anybody—I wouldn't want my mother, my boyfriend, my father, or my family havin' to see me like that. I just think that's not a life; you're not living when it's that bad and I guess it's really scary 'cause I mean when you get to that point and there's really nothin'. And I don't know how long I'll have to live like that, so that's scary. . . . It's not always easy living with it on a daily basis. Especially when it's like movies on TV and then you see people dying, and you're just wondering if that's gonna be you.

Respondents who tried to maintain active lifestyles, specifically work roles, worried about the long-term health consequences of taking on too many responsibilities. Donna, for example, is concerned about the effects of HIV on her health. Her job as a nurses' assistant is physically demanding, and Donna realizes the toll that pushing herself has on her health:

> Sometimes I'm not up to par like I should be. And like I had Saturday, Sunday, Monday, Tuesday off. I didn't get out of bed until Tuesday. I cook something, eat it right in bed, watch TV, pamper myself [because] I know I'm losing a lot of energy. Plus my immune system is kinda being overworked, so when I get home I take good care of myself. I take a shower, and all the bubbles and then I rest. It strains me. Sometimes I get dry

heaves. I get hot and cold flashes. I'm lookin' at my color and I can see my color gettin' a little gray. I'm not up to par; I'm really not up to par like I should be.

When asked how her doctors and other health care professionals describe her health, Donna reported that just two months prior to her interview her physician informed her that her health was deteriorating: "That's what they told me: it's gettin' progressively worse, my condition. And boy, I cried, I cried, and I cried! And then I said, 'Do you think it could be from me workin'?' 'Cause I know really that's the reason, 'cause I go like a bat out of hell." When asked if this decline affected the way she feels about herself, Donna noted that a change in her physical appearance will indeed be bothersome and lead to a negative sense of self:

> Well, if I [looked sick] I would have a low, very low self-esteem. But you know, the *look*. I mean I don't care about the sick, I mean [people] don't know you're sick but they know the look, that look. I'm worried about *that look!* That's the thing. One of my stepbrothers, he died of the same thing and he had marks all over his face, and I worry about that too.

Although individuals with HIV/AIDS are living longer due to early detection and new highly active antiretroviral therapies, these women are well aware that they will die prematurely. Not surprisingly, then, a common thread running through these women's narratives is their anticipatory grief for inevitable losses, including their health, physical appearance, and life ambitions (Dane 1991; Martin and Dean 1993). Anticipatory grief may be beneficial in that it allows for individuals to psychologically prepare for their impending death (Dane 1991; Martin and Dean 1993; Krohn 1998; Riley 1983).

Financial Insecurity

Poverty is a very real concern for many women with HIV infection (Jenkins and Coons 1996; Lather and Smithies 1997; Lee 1995; Ward 1993). For women who are relatively healthy, or at least not functionally impaired, the physiological aspects of HIV/AIDS often take a backseat to the more pressing, immediate issues of survival. When asked what they need most immediately, most respondents cited money as their most urgent need. As already noted, financial stress was a problem for many women in the study long before they contracted HIV infection. For those who were not poor, HIV and ill health posed a threat to their socioeconomic status. Of those who were more likely to worry about their financial well-being, none had partners to help contribute to their living expenses. They were also less likely to have intravenous drug-use histories (67 percent versus 33 percent of women who have intravenous drug histories). Respondents with drug-use histories may be more accustomed to dealing with poverty because they grew up in poorer communities and/or they spent much of their income to support their drug addictions. Women who were diagnosed with HIV infection seven or more years prior to the study were more likely to note this concern than those diagnosed more recently (67 percent and 33 percent, respectively). These women likely have seen their financial resources dwindle more quickly, as they have been surviving longer on less income and have spent more on personal and medical needs.

Medical and treatment costs, loss of employment, single motherhood, and divorce are all scenarios that compound financial difficulties. Lisa, for instance, was having trouble making ends meet, which was exacerbated by her ex-husband not paying child support:

> Now [my financial situation] sucks. Like this apartment, I only pay one-third because they have some program where they have like so many slots for people with the virus or people that have substance-abuse problems or people that were battered. . . . I get disability. I don't get SSI because I did work for all those years. [My daughter] also gets a check under my disability, and if I pass away before she's eighteen she'll still get it. So I'm just gonna try again. I just called the Department of Revenue to try and get child support, but he fought me for years and years and years, so it's not gonna be any different this time. It's just another fight. So financially, yeah, it really has [affected me].

Women such as Lisa are more concerned with trying to make ends meet and securing public assistance than they are with the physiological aspects of HIV/AIDS. For instance, earning about $550 a month as a nursing assistant and living paycheck to paycheck, Donna runs her own and her daughter's household:

I'm just trying to get to the third of the month, so I can complete all my bills and then I'll be so more comfortable, you know? I can relax a little. But I been takin' care of my house, my daughter's house, and it's gettin' a little much, you know? . . . She don't work, and then the three kids get welfare. But she wasn't getting her SSI; all she was gettin' was the welfare so she wouldn't even have enough to make it, so I had to pay her bills last month, pay my bills and her bills. I lost ten pounds [in] three months.

Kristen does not spend a great deal of time dwelling on her illness. In fact, she makes a concerted effort not to think about it. She cannot put it out of her mind completely, however, because since she quit her job she is forced to live on a smaller income:

It comes when I'm lacking money, because I was making a very good salary and I was doing really good. That's when it comes. . . . that's really the only time that I really get depressed is when . . . I don't have any money.

THE PERCEIVED SIGNIFICANCE OF GENDER

Recent research on women and HIV/AIDS has contributed greatly to our understanding of the differential experiences of people with HIV/AIDS rooted in socially constructed gender differences. Given the increased attention to gender as a central analytic category, the extent to which women with HIV/AIDS perceive their experiences as "gendered" was of particular interest in this study. Responses to the question, "Do you think your life would be any different if you were a man with HIV infection?" were brief, even among women who generally gave lengthy, detailed answers to questions. The apparent novelty of the question clearly took some women aback, amused some women, and interested others. In all, half of the respondents felt that gender did not really matter or they could not see how gender would matter. For example, Michelle said, "I have no idea. I mean do I think they're treated any different? I don't really think so. I think it's the same stigma no matter what." Geraldine said facetiously, "I don't know what I'd be as a man, you know what I mean? I don't know what kind of a guy I'd be, if I'd be funny and insane like I am now or if I'd be more serious. Guys are weird. I don't have an answer for that."

Some women thought the question itself was absurd. As Dawn said, "I don't know. That's a funny question. I'll have a sex change and find out." Gina said, "I mean of course if I was a man it would be different, but not because of HIV." Heather's response was typical of women who suspected gender may matter, but who are not sure exactly how: "Well, I never thought about that. I suppose in some ways it would be a little different, I'm just trying to think [of how]. I never really thought about [it]. I'm sure in some ways it has to be different."

Respondents were fairly evenly split in terms of whether they perceived HIV/AIDS to be a more trying illness for women or for men. Of those who expressed that living with HIV is more difficult for women (28 percent), two were quick to note the influence of traditional gender role expectations on women's reactions to their situations. For example, Alicia felt that women would be less likely to abandon their children when their hardships became insurmountable: "I think it's harder on women, especially if she has kids. That's what I would say, how the women have all the problems but the man can just get up and go."

A few women pointed out that men with HIV/AIDS have more resources available to them, such as support groups. As Stephanie and Pat said, respectively:

> I guess there would be more support groups because there's more men infected. Like I hear about the men's support group, and they'd say, "Oh, there's like fifty people in it." I'd be going, "Well, God, there's like five in ours."

> They do more for gay men than they do for women. The [AIDS] project [is] always havin' everything for gay men; that's all you ever hear, gay men and their problems. You never hear anything about gay women, nothin' for them, or even straight women. I guess I wouldn't mind bein' a man 'cause I could get more help, you know?

In addition to the availability of formal services, Julia feels that the gay community in general is more supportive. Julia seriously pondered the question, and after careful thought came to the conclusion that men have more social support:

'Cause [for] the heterosexual women, especially my age, it's scary. I mean there are women that I'm aware of that still don't tell anybody they have this disease, they just sit there in their houses alone with it. The gay community is much more accepting because they've been living with it longer.

Marie was quick to point out that the situation for women is "completely different" because "they do more studies on men."

About the same number of respondents (23 percent) felt that it would probably be more difficult if they were men living with HIV/AIDS. Hillary has taken part in many studies and was used to discussing many of the topics raised, but in reply to this question she said, "I don't know. You know, that's a question that nobody's ever asked me. I never thought about it." She continued by noting that it may be more difficult for men to cope because socially constructed norms of masculinity make it harder for them to express their emotions. Using her prison support group as an example, Hillary said:

Take one of my inmates and his life is one way, take a man who has a family and a job, a real life out here and say maybe from sexual indiscretion gets infected, changes his whole life. And because he's the breadwinner and everything, it might make a big difference. They say men can't show their emotions because then they're like a wimp, they're less of a man, they've gotta maintain the macho image. . . . You need to be able to show feelings, but how do you show feelings where you have to be a tough guy, in prison? . . . [Men] don't have the luxury a woman has of being softer. Yet I think, and I shared this with my inmates, that if you can cry and you can show affection and love, and you can say, "I'm hurting" and "I need help," and you can show tears, you're more of a man than one who can't. And they were like, whoa! And then one said, "Boy, it's nice to get a woman's perspective on this, but we still have to maintain a facade around here."

Similarly, Debra feels that maintaining a masculine facade precludes men from expressing themselves and talking openly about their experiences. She offered a stereotypical distinction between straight and gay men, alleging that gay men are less affected by gender-based social norms:

> Gays, I feel, are more open and more apt to talk about things, and they're usually more intelligent, I find. And straight men have this ego, where gay men are able to put aside their ego. And I think the concentrations aren't as big in ego as they are artistically or on self-development. That's how I feel.

Related to conceptions of masculinity, the stereotype of men being in greater control than women was reflected in Jessica's response: "If anything, being HIV positive and being a woman is better than being a man because a man's supposed to have the image of having their shit together, where women have a tendency not to always have their shit together."

Perhaps stemming from the fact that women give birth and are more likely to seek medical attention, some women maintained that men are the "weaker" sex and hence less able to deal with the physical aspects of HIV/AIDS. For instance, Carmen said:

> I think men can't deal with it. . . . I think they're very wimpy toward the situation. Because my kids' father, he says he wouldn't be able to deal with it, he wouldn't. . . . They get a toothache and they get hysterical, or if they catch a cold they—they whine, you know?

Kristen tersely replied, "They're more [like] babies than women are."

Approximately half of the women in this study consider gender to be salient to their experiences of living with HIV infection. Interestingly, rather than expounding on the connection between gender and the issues or adaptive challenges they identified, they approached the question in terms of which would be worse or more difficult: being a man with HIV infection or a woman with the virus. Although not readily evident to them, they drew on ingrained social constructions of gender to arrive at their conclusions, often speaking not to their unique experiences but to the typical ways in which men's and women's lives and personalities differ.

The other women's reactions to the significance of gender are very similar to respondents in Miller and Kaufman's (1996) study of spousal caregiving for persons with dementia. These authors asked their respondents about the role of gender in caregiving and noted that many thought the question was "stupid" or that they simply did not know how to answer such a question.

Not surprisingly, many women did not explicitly highlight the role of gender in shaping their experiences of living with HIV infection. The social place of many of these women precludes critical gender consciousness. Immediate everyday life concerns, such as economic survival, child care, and substance-abuse problems, form these women's realities. Thus, larger, more abstract issues of power differentials and equity are often not within these women's purview. Rather, as Lorber (1994) notes, the ingrained nature of gender results in its seemingly subtle operation. Indeed, although some of the respondents in this study have gained a greater social consciousness through their activist efforts, many have not been exposed to such vehicles. Clearly, whether readily apparent or not, women's lives and senses of selves are shaped by gender. As will be discussed in Chapter 6, gender expectations, specifically caregiving for young children and infirm adults, are central to some women's experiences.

WOMEN'S UNIQUE EXPERIENCES AND NEEDS

Even if women do not necessarily point to gender differences in general terms, they face specific problems that are clearly gender based. The development and implementation of tailored interventions demand a clear understanding of the ways in which women experience HIV infection and the stressors women face (Goggin et al. 2001; Semple et al. 1993). This analysis suggests that managing rejection and stigma, establishing intimate relationships, dealing with death and dying, and financial survival are primary concerns for women living with HIV/AIDS.

Women's responses to rejection and stigma are consistent with other research regarding seropositive and other ill populations (e.g., Goggin et al. 2001; Schneider and Conrad 1980). As noted, women who do not have a significant other, women who have intravenous drug-use histories, and women who have been living with HIV/AIDS for long periods of time may be especially vulnerable to rejection. People with HIV/AIDS in other studies have avoided stigma by concealing their illness, practicing strategic disclosure, altering their social networks, educating others about HIV/AIDS, and presenting themselves as functioning, productive individuals (Weitz 1991). Similarly, the stigmatized nature of HIV/AIDS has led the women discussed in this text to avoid social situations, such as dating, in which they may have to disclose their status. Others managed by learning more about their illness and becoming involved in HIV/AIDS networks. Although societal reactions to HIV have improved over the course of the epidemic, HIV/AIDS remains a largely misunderstood, stigmatized illness. Although nondisclosure of seropositivity may work well for these women in the short term, it will become more difficult to hide their status as their illness progresses; failing health and physical changes will make hiding AIDS an infeasible approach.

Forming and/or maintaining social and intimate relations is key to women's sense of themselves as women and, hence, their quality of life. In fact, of those respondents who were not at the time of the study involved in an exclusive intimate relationship, 70 percent noted the difficulty of meeting or disclosing their seropositive status to potential mates. This concern was especially troubling for women without a significant other and for women who have not used intravenous drugs. This is not particularly surprising given that women without drug-use histories have not had to contend with serious barriers to relationships such as drug addiction.

Other social roles, such as that of a worker, have not been central in many of these women's lives and hence did not surface as important issues. Similarly, establishing intimate relationships is not as central in the literature concerning gay men with HIV/AIDS. Heterosexual women in another study, for instance, were much more likely than gay male respondents to worry about others and relationship losses (Jenkins and Coons 1996). This may be so, in part, because gay men are more likely to encounter potential partners who are active in the AIDS community and hence more knowledgeable about the disease. This would foster greater acceptance of infected individuals. In addition, they may be more likely to enter into more power-balanced relationships than do women with HIV. Women often lack power and independence and enter, or remain in, unhealthy or violent relationships. Women's difficulty negotiating safe sex with their male partners underscores this fact (Fullilove et al. 1990; Holland et al. 1990; Persson 1994; Somlai et al. 1998). These results should not undermine the difficulties gay men may encounter in disclosing their status and forming relationships, but rather it should emphasize the extent of the problem for women. Women's marked concern regarding the difficulty of forming intimate ties as well as their concerns about rejection points to the importance of social networks for seropositive women.

Some of women's primary concerns may well change over the course of their illness. Financial insecurity is, for most, an enduring problem—present before, and exacerbated by, HIV infection. Stigma will also likely continue to be a primary feature of HIV-positive women's lives. In addition, as they become symptomatic or develop AIDS, sickness and decline will pose new difficulties. Indeed, disease progression engenders tremendous losses of self-esteem and feelings of hopelessness.

Despite the problems and concerns that these women face, they are not without agency, and they have found ways to help mitigate the threat to social status and sense of self caused by their uncertain, stigmatizing illness. The following chapter examines the primary ways in which women cope with HIV/AIDS and discusses how their repair work has affected the ways in which they view their lives and selves.

Chapter 4

Toward Legitimation: Coping with HIV/AIDS

Despite the disruption caused by HIV infection, respondents sought to put their lives back together and to establish narrative coherence. A central part of establishing a coherent sense of self is that of normalizing, in which individuals strive to maintain participation in previously occupied social roles (Becker 1997). This chapter addresses two research questions: How do women repair the disruption caused by their diagnosis and restore their sense of identities? That is, how do women integrate HIV/AIDS into their lives and establish or maintain participation in important social roles (e.g., parent, worker, lover, friend)? What are the limits to women's coping strategies? In addressing these questions, women's primary strategies for dealing with the disruption caused by HIV and reconstructing their identities are presented.

COPING WITH HIV/AIDS: A BRIEF REVIEW OF THE LITERATURE

Coping effectively with the disruption caused by HIV infection is crucial to staying as healthy as possible and minimizing psychological sequelae. Stress from HIV-related symptoms and other life stressors, for example, is associated with higher depression test scores (Jenkins and Coons 1996). Further, compared to other chronically ill populations (e.g., people with cancer), people with AIDS tend to exhibit higher levels of morbidity, greater emotional stress, less effectual coping strategies (e.g., denial), and inadequate social support (Grassi et al. 1997).

Research suggests that individuals with HIV/AIDS, similar to those with other diseases, benefit most from problem-focused coping actions (Peterson, Folkman, and Bakeman 1996; Swindells et al. 1999). Research also suggests that emotion-focused coping may lead to greater levels of depression (DeGenova et al. 1994) and poor quality of life (Swindells et al. 1999). Avoidance coping, on the other hand, is associated with more negative emotions and mood states (Siegel, Gluhoski, and Karus 1997; Simoni and Ng 2000), and greater stress (Koopman et al. 2000).

Moneyham et al. (1998) examined the relative effectiveness of active (i.e., seeking social support, managing the illness, and spiritual activities) and passive (i.e., avoidance) coping strategies on the physical symptoms and emotional distress of women with HIV infection. They found that emotional distress decreased with greater use of active coping, controlling for an increase in physical symptoms, suggesting that active coping protects against emotional distress. Similarly, Hart et al. (2000) found that individuals who used denial to cope with their illness reported significantly greater pain severity. Women reported greater pain and higher use of emotion-based coping than did men. These results underscore the potential negative impact of avoidance coping.

In addition to being psychologically unhealthy, avoidance strategies such as denial may also be physiologically harmful. For example, investigating the symptom experience of women with HIV infection, Stevens (1996) found that as women became burdened by symptoms, they sought to protect themselves from allowing HIV to take over their health. Perceiving medical care and compliance with treatment regimens as surrendering to HIV, many acted to avoid these behaviors.

Although more research has examined coping among men with HIV/AIDS, samples comprised of (or including) women suggest that women employ both emotion- and problem-focused coping strategies (e.g., Demi et al. 1997; Moneyham et al. 1998; Siegel, Gluhoski, and Karus 1997; Van-Servellen, Sarna, and Jablonski 1998; Weitz 1991). One of the most visible problem-focused coping strategies is involvement in AIDS activism. Originating from members of the gay rights movement, AIDS activists have been remarkably successful in their efforts to politicize HIV infection, effecting social change and reconstructing biomedical knowledge. AIDS activism has helped reshape the social identities of people with HIV/AIDS, increase federal funding for AIDS research and treatment, and expand access to clinical trials (Bix 1997; Epstein 1995; Wachter 1992). Although emphasis on treatment, in lieu of prevention, has been criticized for neglecting the needs of other HIV/AIDS populations (e.g., injection drug users) (Wachter 1992), the achievements of AIDS activists are undeniable. Although many activist groups may attract, and cater to, the needs of white, middle-upper-class gay men, heterosexual women with HIV/AIDS may also reap the benefits of participation.

Many respondents in Weitz's (1990) sample, for example, managed their illness and concomitant stigma by concealing their illness or through selective disclosure. They distanced themselves from unsupportive friends and family and found support elsewhere, such as in support groups for people with HIV/AIDS. Participation in community organizations and AIDS education was another way in which interviewees coped with HIV infection. As their illness progressed, their coping strategies were less directed at reducing stigma and more directed at managing their symptoms. For example, they put their energies into reevaluating their physical appearances and emphasizing past accomplishments, rather than dwelling on inevitable losses.

Long-term AIDS survivors appear to employ many of the same coping behaviors as do those in the earlier stages of the disease. For example, among Barroso's (1997a) primarily male sample of long-term AIDS survivors, respondents engaged in normalizing behavior (e.g., maintaining one's daily routine), focused on living (e.g., maintaining a positive attitude about one's life and illness), practiced self-care (e.g., abstaining from drugs), renegotiated familial and friendship relations, sought to help others with HIV infection, and triumphed (e.g., transcended their illness via reframing AIDS into a situation over which they had greater control).

In fact, in coping with their disease, many women have come to highlight the positive aspects of being HIV positive, including renewed relationships, newfound values and purpose, greater self-awareness and self-acceptance, and new spiritual connections (Dunbar et al. 1998; Goggin et al. 2001; Moser, Sowell, and Phillips 2001). In addition, HIV infection has led women to reassess their relationships, lifestyles and priorities, which aids them in their coping efforts (Barroso 1997a; Dunbar et al. 1998; Gillman and Newman 1996; Henderson 1992).

WOMEN'S WAYS OF COPING:
REPAIRING DISRUPTED BIOGRAPHIES

The majority of the women in this sample are working HIV infection into their biographies, and many are striving to keep HIV/AIDS from becoming their primary defining characteristic. Clearly, this task is easier for women who are asymptomatic and can ignore or downplay their illness to a certain extent. In addition, those who are on promising new drug therapies, such as protease inhibitors, have come to believe that they can live happy, worthwhile lives. As with respondents in other studies, women in this study employed a variety of styles of repair work. Use of humor, maintaining a positive outlook, better self-care, and stress reduction were employed as ways of coping. As with previous research, (e.g., Jaccard, Wilson, and Radecki 1995), the most common strategies include going public with their illness, joining support groups, seeking or strengthening religious/spiritual ties, establishing positive lifestyles, and avoidance/denial. The first three legitimation styles demonstrate the importance of relational resources (Bury 1982), as they involve group interaction and support. However, in focusing on spirituality and religion, women also tapped cognitive resources (Bury 1982) as they interpreted their illness as ultimately in the hands of a higher power. In doing so, these women were able to gain comfort from the notion that their fate was out of their control. Women who coped with their illness mainly by establishing positive lifestyles did so primarily by seeking material resources. Women who avoided or denied their illness were cognitively reconstructing HIV/AIDS into a minor event, one to which they need not devote much attention or energy.

GOING PUBLIC AND BECOMING AN ACTIVIST

Deciding whom to tell (if anyone at all) and when is a major stressor for individuals with HIV/AIDS (Foley et al. 1994; Semple et al. 1993; Stein and Hanna 1997; Weitz 1991). Women may avoid disclosure for fear of losing custody of their children, being rejected by loved ones, being physically assaulted, and facing discrimination in employment, housing, and/or social services (Carlson et al. 1997; Jenkins and Coons 1996; Kalichman and Catz 2000; Moneyham et al. 1996). Women with substance-abuse histories, who have been rejected from family members prior to contracting HIV infection, may be especially vulnerable to further alienation as they may be seen as responsible for their predicament (Crystal and Schiller 1993; Lawless, Kippax, and Crawford 1996; Schneider 1992). Despite justified fears, many individuals eventually disclose their diagnosis to at least a few people to secure support (Carlson et al. 1997; Gillman and Newman 1996; Lévy et al. 1999). The majority of women in this sample also told others about their illness, particularly family members. In addition to disclosing their diagnosis, some women went a step farther and became active in HIV/AIDS organizations to reshape societal attitudes toward people with HIV/AIDS and to effect social change. Going public as a form of repair was more typical among women who did not have intravenous drug-use histories than it was among women who did have intravenous drug-use histories (71 percent and 29 percent, respectively). This may be because women with intravenous drug-use histories are typically less socially organized than those without drug-use histories, and thus they may be less likely to want to participate in such efforts. In addition, due to their illicit histories, these women may be less well received as public spokespersons. Women who did not contract the virus via needle sharing, for example, are more likely to elicit sympathy from the general public. Women who were not involved in an intimate relationship were also more likely to engage in going public than women who did have a partner (57 percent and 43 percent, respectively). Perhaps in an attempt to protect the family's privacy, partners discourage women from going public. Partners may also coerce women into keeping their diagnosis a secret to maintain privacy. In addition, men who strive to be in control of their lover may see their partner's potentially greater independence and reliance on others as a threat to their dominant position. This strategy was much more typical among women who had been living with HIV for seven or more years (71 percent versus 29 percent of women diagnosed fewer than seven years prior). This may be due, in part, to the fact that women who have had HIV infection for long periods have had more time to incorporate their illness into their biographies and, hence, are more comfortable sharing their experiences. Similarly, women who have survived so long may be more optimistic about their living well with HIV infection and, hence, more willing to tell their stories to the world. In addition, over the years they may have gained more experience with medical and so-

cial service networks and therefore have become more effective outreach people.

As with women with other illnesses, women in this study sought to
lessen the blow of HIV/AIDS on their daily lives. Their involvement
in epidemiological studies and HIV/AIDS organizations no doubt introduced them to avenues for developing problem-focused strategies
(i.e., efforts to change or manage stressors that seem mutable) and
many took advantage of them.

AIDS activism, similar to that of other groups, including women
with breast cancer and persons with mental illness, can have tremendous social impact and personal fulfillment (Batt 1992; Chamberlin
1978; Wachter 1992). On an individual level, Register (1989) called
coming to terms with illness a conversion experience. She writes, "it
alters your outlook on life, reorders your values, changes your behavior, and can leave you with a missionary zeal to aid others in a similar
predicament" (1989:104). Indeed, for some of the respondents in this
study (19 percent), publicly disclosing their HIV status and/or becoming involved in AIDS education and prevention efforts has been
central to repair. The degree to which these respondents went public
varied, but all agreed that disclosure is crucial to healing and to working HIV into their biographies. Many women associated disclosure
with good mental health. For example, Jennifer is very open about
her HIV infection because for her, "secrets are stress," and she feels
that to live a healthy life she must minimize anxiety.

Others initially became involved in helping to educate the public
about HIV/AIDS. Through sharing their knowledge and experiences,
they help themselves to cope. These women developed a sense of
purpose in using their illness experience to help others (Coward
1994). For example, although Laurie is still grappling with disruption
she has come a long way in the six years that she has been living with
HIV infection. When asked how she copes with the virus, she responded:

> I'm getting better at it. I've gotten to the point where if I can help
> another woman realize that it can happen to you, then I do. I've
> been on [local news channels], I used to go speaking at schools,
> try and educate people that it's no longer a gay disease.

Equally important, going public helps garner support from others,
including other women with HIV/AIDS and health care and social

service professionals. This was the case for Lisa, who does not have a supportive familial network. Lisa was diagnosed with HIV infection nine years prior to the study and has since developed AIDS. Following the death of their two-year-old daughter, Marisa, from AIDS, Lisa and her husband's relationship became strained. Blaming her for Marisa's death, he could no longer be in the same room as Lisa, much less be her partner. Following their separation, Lisa found herself alone trying to cope with the loss of her child, the problems of her troubled adolescent daughter, and HIV. For her, going public was a way of securing much-needed emotional support. Lisa now tells her story—of having AIDS and losing a daughter to the virus—to local reporters and television news personalities:

> I started telling people slowly; now I don't care who knows. My husband has a big problem with that—he has a real big problem. But I have been public: I've been on TV, in the paper, and I really don't care. But my daughter doesn't seem to have a problem with it either, I mean, if she had a problem with it then I would not be as vocal, but [I won't stop for] him. I don't even understand. It's like he's ashamed of it. Why is he ashamed of it?

In addition to blaming her for Marisa's death, Lisa's husband also bears a courtesy stigma (Goffman 1963) of being associated with Lisa, because he perceives her as deviant. He is ashamed to have any connection to HIV/AIDS or with anyone infected. Despite her husband's rejection, Lisa is slowly learning to work HIV into her biography and to establish a coherent sense of self. By going public, she is vulnerable to greater alienation. Her involvement, however, has had positive effects. When asked if her participation is therapeutic, she responded: "Yes, definitely, because if I didn't have the support, my family was not supportive." Describing her self-perception over time, she reported that although she still experiences guilt over her daughter's death, the stigma has lessened: "I still have the guilt, but I don't feel—I don't have the sign over my forehead." Thus, by interacting with individuals who convey a genuine, nonjudgmental interest in her experiences and encourage her to share her story, Lisa has been provided the opportunity to incorporate HIV into her life and to rebuild her self-esteem.

Those with supportive informal networks also reap the benefits of public involvement. Sheila, for example, has a very supportive husband who she said helped her cope with HIV and restore her self-esteem. Sheila cannot forget, however, the not-so-distant past when HIV caused her to feel inferior, afraid, and angry. When she was diagnosed she "felt like dirt" and abstained from social involvement. She described how she felt:

> I always used to be one evil, angry person . . . from the time that I found out until the last two years. I was bitter at the whole world. . . . I would always go to work because that's me, I love to work. I'd go to school, take care of my children. But I would deal with people only when I had to.

In addition to receiving informal support, Sheila now is socially active and is involved in HIV/AIDS groups. In fact, she is a cofacilitator of a support group for incarcerated women infected with HIV/AIDS. By sharing her experiences with others, she hopes to help other women in similar situations:

> My goal now is to try to help other people that have this virus and let them know that you can plan for the future—life does go on, not to give up. I've always learned that if you're a fighter you'll be okay. You have to fight and you have to want to live. If you have a lot of negativism, that is a big drawback—and if you carry that anger and that hurt around, that can destroy you. . . .When I finally started accepting the fact and telling people, I felt like a big burden was lifted off of my shoulder. It's like, boy, I can say it and not really be ashamed.

As these excerpts illustrate, Sheila has indeed come a long way since diagnosis and has emerged with a renewed outlook on life and a renewed sense of self. In retrospect, Sheila acknowledges that the virus has helped her to construct a positive sense of self: "I'm glad in a way that I have this virus because it made me a very strong person. It also has made me look at life in a different way. I enjoy everything I do. I enjoy the trees, I enjoy the sun, I mean *everything*." Sheila hopes that other women can gain strength from her fight. In fact, when asked what she could use most at present, Sheila did not make reference to material goods for herself. Rather, she expressed a humanitarian goal of helping others: "To be able to go out and just help every person that is infected, and to reach them."

As previously noted, the fact that Hillary has AIDS does not stop her from devoting time and energy to help others with the virus. She was relieved when she was able to go public with her illness and share her story. In addition to the personal gains, Hillary noted that she is fortunate to be able to go public, to participate in activist causes without the threat of alienating loved ones or threatening her job security:

> By being out there I hope that I'm making it easier for other people. I'm doing it for the ones that can't, because not everybody can [go public]. There's so much to lose. I have the luxury of not losing anything by being public, except somebody that isn't really a friend, and I can live without that. I know I'm doing it for other people, and when I see the effect I'm having—you know, it may not be a big thing, but if I'm making a positive difference in anybody's life, even in a little way, it's so worth it. . . . And I tell all my clients I'm infected; that's one of the first things they learn when they come in. Because I want them to understand that I understand where they're coming from, and what they're living, 'cause I'm living it.

For some women, going public was not an easy, natural response. Gina was not always vocal about women and AIDS. She was so impressed by the pertinent issues that the members of a Massachusetts-based group were tackling, such as guardianship, that she joined the organization. Initially, however, she was reticent about becoming involved in any organized activity:

> For a while I had refused any contact with whatever has to do [with the virus], except going to the doctor and doing my testing and stuff. I didn't want to get involved with nothing concerned with AIDS because I was afraid that I was going to meet people and get attached to people and then these people were gonna die. And it did happen eventually.

Soon Gina realized that her fear of losing friends to HIV/AIDS was standing in her way of helping herself and others. She made a transformation from a recluse of sorts to an activist. In fact, she is critical of those who want public goods and services but are not politically active:

Sometimes I feel like . . . a lot of clients come here only for the money, like they need a check to buy some food or like get in a study just to get some money. Don't get me wrong; that's a good part, but, you know, on the other hand it has to be part of a bigger picture. I guess this disease has had stages. You know, you get to "Why me, what did I do?" And then you get to the point then you have to do something. . . . Unless [you're] part of moving things along, you feel like nothing is gonna change. I found myself saying, "It's pretty stupid that I sit here and complain—this doesn't work, that doesn't work—and do nothing about it." . . . So I really, toward this disease, I guess I got that attitude . . . there are things that you can do.

Respondents who went public are not a homogeneous group; they differ in terms of substance-abuse and sexual histories, socioeconomic status, and availability of informal support. Yet the experience of coming out and publicly disclosing their HIV status has brought them to a similar place in their lives. These women have come to highlight the positive aspects of having HIV/AIDS. An illness, which initially symbolized the end of life, became a source of strength and self-growth.

SUPPORT GROUPS

Subcultures, such as self-help groups, may be an important resource for people coping with illness and disability (Schneider and Conrad 1980). Those dealing with a stigmatized illness can learn practical survival skills from the experiences of others. Research suggests that participation in support groups for people with HIV/AIDS may enhance self-efficacy (Land 1994); reduce social isolation (Land 1994), emotional distress (Kalichman, Sikkema, and Somlai 1996; Kelly et al. 1993), and drug use (Magura et al. 1991); foster greater disclosure of seropositivity status to potential sex partners (Greenberg, Johnson, and Fichtner 1996); increase knowledge of HIV/AIDS illness progression (Jenkins and Coons 1996); and improve attitudes toward condom use (Gupta and Weiss 1993; Magura et al. 1991).

The majority of respondents in this study (nearly 60 percent) were not attending a support group at the time of the interview, but for the women who were involved in groups (42 percent), interaction with other individuals with HIV infection was crucial to their repair process. Most of the respondents (83 percent) who credited support groups with helping them cope did not have intravenous drug-use histories (versus 17 percent of women who had intravenous drug-use histories). Similar to engaging in the "going public" strategy, it is likely that intravenous drug users are less willing to become involved in organized groups. In addition, women who did not have a partner were more likely to be active in HIV/AIDS groups than women involved in an intimate relationship (86 percent and 14 percent, respectively). Although not as public as participating in AIDS prevention and education efforts, support groups do entail disclosure of personal information. As such, partners may view support groups as a threat to familial privacy. The length of time women have been living with HIV did not appear to make a difference in women's participation; women diagnosed over seven years prior to this study and those diagnosed more recently were equally likely to be support group members.

Sharing their experiences in a supportive atmosphere fostered greater understanding of the disease and a more positive sense of self. Unlike the women who went public, many of these women do not disclose their HIV status to everyone. Although they do not want their serostatus to be public knowledge, they do not want to go through their illness alone, and they have found support in a confidential and, for the most part, nonjudgmental environment.

Support groups for people with HIV/AIDS and drug addicts provide a forum for women to speak openly about their needs and fears. Perhaps most important, at least initially, these groups show women that they are not alone. It is easy for women with HIV/AIDS, especially those who were socially isolated prior to diagnosis, to feel as if they are the only people struggling with HIV infection. As Thalia said: "I know nobody. It's like you feel like you're the only person on the planet [with HIV infection]. I feel like I'm the only person."

Carmen demonstrates this point well. As discussed in Chapter 2, when Carmen found out she was HIV positive, she "wanted to die" and attempted suicide shortly after her diagnosis. Joining a substance-abuse support group changed Carmen's view of people with HIV/AIDS and assured her that she was not alone. Of the drug treatment center, she said:

There was a lot of people there that were positive and they were living like normal people. So after awhile I got used to it, being that everybody there was mostly positive. So with them I felt like I was normal, they helped me to deal with it.

The normalizing experience offered by group involvement is, in fact, the most positive aspect of participation voiced by these women. As with Carmen, Becky became so depressed at times that she thought she would be better off dead: "I've wanted to give up. I've hoped that this disease would wipe me out. When I got sick or when I was extremely depressed and sick, I'd say to myself, 'Well, I'm gonna die anyway.'" She further described herself in those early years as "very withdrawn and ashamed." Becky explained that over the seven years of living with HIV prior to this study, she has come to think very differently about herself and her ability to live a full life. By sharing her experiences with others and hearing their stories, Becky has learned to better deal with her illness:

By watching other people with it deal with it . . . like you deal with life. My outlook today is that I have a life, period. Just like anyone else with or without [HIV], I can live with it. If someone would have told me that I was gonna have this disease . . . I would've said, "Ha, ha, ha." . . . You finally realize when you're faced with a situation you don't think you ever could deal with and you don't want to deal with it, [but] by working with that you build your self-esteem, and education is number one, key. And talking about it—I don't mean with people on the street who I don't know—but just being up front with a group that you can share it with.

Becky reported that her greatest lesson from participation in twelve-step drug programs and support groups for people with HIV/AIDS is that she is "not totally powerless over [her] life." For women who fear the physical and psychosocial losses associated with HIV/AIDS, empowerment is crucial to living full and happy lives, and clearly an important part of legitimation.

The women in this sample who went public appear to be coping with their illness very well. They do not claim to be experts on living with the virus, nor have they exhausted the benefits of support group participation. Lisa participates in a group for women with HIV as well as a group for parents of HIV-infected children, which she joined when Marisa, her daughter, was still alive. Talking about Marisa's death in the parents' group was very difficult for Lisa. She noted, however, that had she not interacted with other parents going through a similar experience, she would not have made as much progress as she had in terms of alleviating the guilt associated with Marisa's death.

Some women in this study voiced concern that participation in support groups for people with HIV/AIDS may place the condition at the center of their lives, rather than deeming it merely one component of their identity, albeit an important one. These comments further illustrate their quest for normalcy as they strive to balance their ill, "deviant" selves with their healthy, normal selves. Feeling bombarded with information about and experiences of living with HIV infection counteracts women's efforts to feel like normal people (i.e., people who do not have a stigmatized condition). As Jennifer, a support group member of ten years, explained:

> Every now and then I take a break. I'll take a month or two break every now and then because I feel like I'm inundated with AIDS. So sometimes I do have to take that break. A lot of people, they just overload themselves and they wanna help everybody and they do this and do that and then they burn out.

Carolyn also feels the need at times to distance herself from other people with HIV infection. Although she values the organization and friends she has made there, she noted that groups can be somewhat disheartening:

> I don't even want to be around an HIV-positive person who's constantly whining. I like to turn the depression thing around, I like to be around people who can do that. I do pretty good for myself, enough suffering is enough. Whatever it takes, get your mind on something else. I usually end up saying, "Oh, the hell with this. The hell with it all." Because if you dwell on it you'll drive yourself crazy. I get it over with, do my squealin', unplug the phone, stay in the house for a week, whatever it takes, and then get over it.

Indeed, the fear of HIV/AIDS becoming one's defining characteristic is troublesome. Becky, for example, also worries that by tending too closely to living with HIV/AIDS her identity will be subsumed by her illness. She said: "I am not about HIV. It's not like my name is Becky and I have HIV and AIDS. It's not like that, you know?"

To summarize, in coping with the disease, many of these women mobilized new resources (Carricaburu and Pierret 1995). To this end, they often joined support groups, and some began facilitating groups and speaking publicly about their experiences. By participating in support groups and other vehicles by which they could share their experiences, they obtained information about HIV/AIDS, garnered social support, and gained respect and acceptance from esteemed others, e.g., health care professionals. This last point is extremely important, as for some, particularly women with substance-abuse histories, this was the first time they had received this degree of positive attention from their health care providers. Women spoke very highly of the organizations from which they were recruited and were likewise positive about the professionals who served them. Support from health care professionals may be especially important for women lacking supportive informal networks.

Many gay men with HIV/AIDS, at least in urban areas, have access to a community of support. Similarly, participation in support groups and/or HIV/AIDS organizations provides role models for women and underscores the fact that they are not alone, and perhaps helps to alleviate social isolation (Henderson 1992). In addition, involvement in the AIDS community may foster more healthy, effective coping strategies, and in turn, lead to better adaptation (Leserman, Perkins, and Evans 1992; Sosnowitz 1995). As HIV/AIDS continues to increase among heterosexual women, "a parallel community for HIV+ women is developing; women's support groups are an ideal strategy for building this community" (Lather and Smithies 1997:183).

However, unlike most of the women interviewed for this study, many women with HIV/AIDS are not well linked to health and social services and may not have any knowledge of how to become involved in such groups. Further, if there is not a group/organization in their communities, women may be hesitant to join groups in outlying areas. The women in this study who were from Georgia, for example, explained that their group was convenient, and this meant that they did not have to commute to Atlanta to be involved. The psychological hurdles of attending a support group, including fear of exposure, fear of seeing very ill people, and an erosion of denial, may also preclude one's involvement (Lather and Smithies 1997).

Women are also less likely than their male counterparts to have HIV-positive friends. In a qualitative study of women with HIV/AIDS, for example, only 39 percent identified at least one close friend who was also HIV positive, whereas studies of gay men demonstrate much higher percentages of HIV-positive friends (Semple et al. 1993). Similarly, among this sample, with the exclusion of fellow support group members, approximately 37 percent of respondents were close to another person with HIV infection, most typically lovers and friends. Thus, women may not know or meet other infected women with whom to share their experiences and obtain support. Again, support groups may well fill this need. Indeed, there is evidence that although many women are initially leery of joining support groups, they later become a valuable asset to women coping with HIV infection (Jenkins and Coons 1996).

Same-sex groups are an important source of solidarity for those who are often isolated and stigmatized by HIV (Littlewood 1994). Although support groups for infected men welcome women, some women may feel uncomfortable and alienated. Indeed, the virus does not offset gender and lifestyle differences and women may find the discussions in men's groups unrelated to their experiences and concerns (Land 1994; Lather and Smithies 1997). Further, some women may be uncomfortable in groups discussing male homosexuality.

We may add race and class differences here as well. Indeed, some of the women in this sample found it hard to relate to other women in their support groups with drug-addiction histories or stories of racism and discrimination. Some women, such as Stephanie, may have a hard time connecting with other women with HIV/AIDS due to class and lifestyle differences.

SPIRITUALITY

Organized religion or, more typically, spiritual involvement plays an important role in the lives of many terminally ill people. HIV diagnosis is often an impetus to renew or strengthen spiritual or religious ties. Indeed, the connection between spirituality and wellness and health care practices has received considerable recent attention by social scientists and health care providers alike (e.g., Avants, Warburton, and Margolin 2001; Carr and Morris 1996; do-Rozario 1997;

Hall 1997; Millison 1995; Nolan and Crawford 1997; Pace and Stables 1997; Stolley and Koenig 1997; Ventis 1995). The importance of spirituality in coping with HIV/AIDS has also been noted (e.g., Barroso 1997a; Coward 1994; Kaplan, Marks, and Mertens 1997; Mellins et al. 1996; Sowell et al. 2000; Woods et al. 1999). Religious and/or spiritual activities are an important resource for maintaining psychological well-being—by helping to reduce stress, sustain a positive outlook, and maintain higher quality of life, for example.

Further, despite the fact that "religious teachings have been identified as a facilitator of intolerance toward people with HIV or those in HIV risk groups," religious organizations have also been key players in grassroots advocacy for people with HIV/AIDS and instrumental in implementing peer support and counseling programs (Jenkins 1995:132). Further, some research suggests that religious and spiritual coping have been more effective than other methods (e.g., problem solving and interpersonal support) in ameliorating illness-related distress by helping respondents reinterpret their situations and focus on the positive aspects of what may appear tragic (Jenkins 1995).

Among the women in this study's sample, spirituality appeared to be an important coping strategy for those without a partner than for those who have a significant other (63 percent and 37 percent, respectively). Women without a partner may have a greater need for support, and spirituality may help fill this void. Similarly, intravenous drug-use histories appear to be a factor; that is, of those noting the importance of spirituality, 63 percent have never used intravenous drugs (versus 37 percent who have intravenous drug-use histories). Perhaps women with substance-abuse histories are less likely to have formed religious or spiritual ties in their lives before learning they were HIV positive and, hence, are less likely to establish such ties after diagnosis. Spirituality was also more typical among women who had been HIV positive for seven or more years than it was among women who were diagnosed fewer than seven years prior to this study (75 percent and 25 percent, respectively). Women who had been living with HIV for long periods of time may feel sickness approaching more rapidly and seek spirituality as an ultimate coping strategy.

From the moment Donna was diagnosed with HIV and "the Lord took it all off [her] shoulders," her faith has helped her cope. Donna often experiences physical fatigue and emotional distress; she has very little money and she helps support her adult children, getting little help in return. Her strong faith helps alleviate this stress: "I don't get too stressed out because I know God up above will take care of it all. Sometimes, you kinda lack that thought. And then it kinda depresses you."

Donna learned about the power of faith the hard way—when she was struggling with cancer. It was not clear whether Donna's cancer had gone into remission or whether the neoplasm was removed without metastasizing, but whatever the case, she believes God healed her:

> 'Cause like [in] 1986 I had colon cancer, and I went down. I couldn't walk, couldn't talk. I was just like a little vegetable. But then they cured me, so I just leave it up to God. I'm not gonna worry about stuff like that. You just care more about God because when he calls your number, if you're sick or not, you're going.

Her experience with cancer influenced her view toward HIV in that she was not interested in her prognosis. Donna explained that she is forthright about her beliefs and tells her physicians that the less information she receives, the better:

> I mean, you know, if I'm dying tomorrow, please don't tell me. Just let it happen naturally. . . . You don't know what's going on in your life that's gonna take you tomorrow, so don't say I'm goin' tomorrow. Doctors really think they can determine when you're goin', have a good idea, but only the man upstairs knows it. I know you're doin' your job, but just don't tell me.

As Donna suggested, spirituality can be a critical resource when facing mortality. A belief in an afterlife can be very comforting, alleviating some of the fear of dying. Geraldine explained how her religious convictions have helped her deal with HIV and death:

> I'm not afraid. I have like a really good relationship with God and we're like buddies. And if He said tomorrow, "Go," I'd be like, "I'm leaving tomorrow, see you, it's been real nice but I'm going to a nice little place." But I'm not gonna get a warning . . . I don't even think of [getting sick]. No, if it's gonna come, it's gonna come, you know?

Living with HIV for nine years at the time of this study, Geraldine is asymptomatic and has not had any major HIV-related health problems. Given her length of seropositivity, however, she realizes that her chances of becoming symptomatic and/or progressing to AIDS are high. In an effort to combat decline, Geraldine took part in a healing ceremony at her church about six weeks prior to participating in this project. Recalled Geraldine:

> They had this thing at church, the anointing of the sick. . . . I got up and [Father Michael] was on the altar . . . so I went right up to him and he put his hands on my little head and he talked to God like by himself, you know? And then he got this stuff and he said some things and he put like a cross on my head and then he put one in one hand and one in the other hand, he put my two hands together and it meant so much because like he knew why I was there, you know what I mean? He knows what I'm all about. And I'll tell you the weirdest thing, my luck and my life has turned totally around since that.

Their families or friends introduced some respondents to religion. Most of these women were not particularly religious before being diagnosed, but HIV, coupled with their association with religious others, sparked their involvement. Sheila's husband, Bill, for instance, is very active in their church. He prides himself on speaking and living the word of God. In fact, Bill himself discussed his religious beliefs during his interview for this study. He firmly believes that through strong faith in God anything is possible, including a cure for HIV/AIDS. Sheila is not as observant as Bill, but she reported that his strong religious convictions are starting to rub off on her:

> My parents brought me up in the church and I never used to go to church every Sunday, but when I felt that spiritual need I would pop in. But it's something that you just have in your heart, it's just there. But now, 'cause he's very, very religious . . . and since I met him I go more. . . . He believes that if you have faith [then] God will heal everybody and anybody, that faith is strong enough.

Although her faith is a source of consolation, Sheila also feels torn between her husband's religious beliefs and her health care providers' recommendations:

They started me on AZT, 3TC, and I took it for a month and then decided I can't. Then I had to deal with my husband. I come home with these drugs, he's like, "What are you doing?" And he says to me, "Honey, you know I love you." And he says, "We gotta have faith." I'm like, "But, baby, I have these kids. I want to live long enough to at least see my kids." I want to live long enough to see my kids grow up, after that I don't care what happens to me because I lived my life.

Although religious and medical doctrine need not conflict, Bill's beseeching has put Sheila in an awkward and possibly dangerous position as she feels compelled to place her health solely in God's hands. Despite a dropping T-cell count and increasing viral load, Sheila stopped taking her medications. In recounting her conversation with her physician, she said:

To me, it's like I feel fine, I feel good. I get tired because I have a busy lifestyle—I work, I take care of this house, I take care of my family; what person would not get tired? Then the point comes back up or the feeling comes back up—they say they can make you live an extra five years but I know deep down in my heart that no drug or no one can make you live an extra five or ten years. I believe when God says your time is up, your time is up, I don't care what your takin'. So that's where I am now in my life. I believe, why make yourself feel terrible when you really don't have to? But I know that if I don't try to take these pills like I should that then my count will go down, and that I'm the one that has to live with that feeling of "Did I do everything that I could to make myself stay well?" It's hard. And, like I said, I think my thing is I don't like to be poppin' almost sixteen to seventeen pills a day.

As illustrated in this excerpt, Sheila realizes the gamble she is taking with her health by going off her medications. She lived with HIV infection for eight years and has developed AIDS. On one hand, she intelligently speaks about her health and its likely trajectory. However, by attributing her fatigue to her work and familial responsibilities, Sheila is able to justify (to herself and others) her decision to seek help through God rather than biomedicine. Sheila and Bill think of their congregation as family, thus the response of the church community to her illness was of utmost importance to them. Sheila is relieved that her church community knows she has AIDS and she values the support they give her. She is hoping that the support from her family and congregation will be enough.

Spiritual involvement may also provide alternative therapies that help people with HIV infection cope. Carolyn has reaffirmed her religious ties and has returned to activities in which she engaged as a youth, particularly meditation. In addition, Carolyn reported that her new age church is akin to a support group in that they accept and treat their members with love and respect regardless of background or lifestyle:

> They do meditation, which I never thought about, but even as a child I did that. I mean, I'd go out in the hills—I lived in the country—sit under the tree and think. So this church is doing that. And they remind everybody that everyone in this world is equal—man, woman, black or white. And they don't care if you're homosexual, you are welcome in this church. It's not our place to judge these people, and they're loved just as much as you are—that is my philosophy, so I love this church.

Looking at Carolyn, one would never suspect that she has a fatal infection. Because she does not look sick she is able to pass as healthy and does not need to disclose her status to members of her church. Although she suspects that they would not ostracize her, she can only speculate as to what their reaction would be; thus, although she draws inspiration and emotional support from her participation in the new age church, they may not be a solid source of support in the long run.

Religious faith offers not only consolation but also redemption. Having a life-threatening disease certainly brings mortality to the fore. Facing death, one may seek forgiveness for past sins. This is true of Rachel who found herself praying more frequently since her diagnosis. Although she is hesitant to credit HIV infection as the impetus for increased prayer, she would not discredit it either:

> I do pray a lot now, maybe it's because of the condition I'm in. I don't know, maybe I would have prayed otherwise, maybe not. [I pray], "Forgive me, forgive me," you know. I try not to hurt anybody, [but] I've hurt people, not intentionally. I have, and I felt like shit about it.

In discussing her support systems, Heather said, "it's God above all, then medically it's [my doctor], and emotionally it's my husband." Heather's Catholic upbringing, though, did not offer her a guarantee that she would go to heaven. Her roommate, Susan, however, appeared to have the spiritual security Heather craved. Desperately seeking assurance that she would be in a better place after she died, Heather turned to Susan for guidance:

> Well, needless to say when I found out about having the HIV virus I didn't know how long I had to live, and I thought I want whatever she has because I don't know, and she knows, and I need to know. I remember I just said, "Susan, I need to have what you have, I need to know that I'm gonna go to heaven, not just hope I'm gonna be good enough to get in."

A prayer Susan gave her proved to be a transcendent experience; it provided Heather with the strength to face HIV/AIDS and reconstruct a positive sense of self:

> She gave me this prayer, and I went up in my bedroom—I remember it like it was yesterday. This was the turning point in my whole [life] as far as feeling better. I remember saying that prayer with my heart of hearts and really not just saying the words, you know how we can tend to pray, repitiously; I was saying those words with every bit of feeling I had in me. I wanted this salvation! And then I went to sleep and the next morning I went to work. . . . I'm working through the morning and everything and I was feeling very good, and this was pre-protease inhibitors and I'm feeling really good. And since then my spiritual life has progressed. My husband and I go to a Bible church, so we're learning a lot. I truly believe that it's through God that the scientists and the researchers have developed the protease inhibitors and all these drugs that we have now. So all the glory is His.

By embracing a religion that offers her a more genuine connection with God, Heather believes that her renewed faith, coupled with her medical treatment, will see her through her illness and help her cope with death and dying.

Spirituality offered these women emotional support and strength. A couple of respondents believed their strong faiths could offer intervention and treatment (e.g., Geraldine and Sheila). Participating in the more social aspects of their spirituality, such as attending services, also provided a safe social environment in which women could gain a sense of belonging.

Although spirituality is an emotion-focused strategy and, in and of itself, a less effective way of managing illness, it is clearly helping women to cope psychologically. Although not clearly demonstrated in this sample, religious involvement may be especially important for black and Latina women (Sosnowitz 1995). Strong religious ties, such as that among many Latinos and in the Catholic Church, have been criticized for hindering productive responses to the threat of HIV/AIDS. The traditional handling of sensitive topics, such as homosexuality and gender, have posed great barriers to AIDS education and prevention (Sosnowitz 1995). Given the importance many women assign to spirituality as a coping mechanism, however, clinicians must be careful not to dismiss it as an illegitimate or devalued resource in helping women adapt to HIV infection when introducing them to other methods. Rather, the strengths and shortcomings of religion as a way of dealing with HIV/AIDS should be discussed.

ESTABLISHING POSITIVE LIFESTYLES

Other women in this sample coped with their illness by establishing and maintaining healthy lifestyles. Putting their energies into healthier living (e.g., better eating habits, exercise, and abstaining from illicit drug use) became part of their daily activities. Women who did not have partners were more likely than women with partners to make positive lifestyle changes (60 percent and 40 percent, respectively). Partners, especially those who minimize the seriousness of HIV infection and/or are active drug users, may consciously or inadvertently discourage women from establishing healthier lifestyles. Another possibility may be that women involved in romantic relationships are putting greater energy into their partners' well-being and tending less to their own needs. Also, more of the women (67 percent) employing this strategy did not have intravenous drug-use histories (versus 33 percent of women who had drug-use histories). This is probably due to the fact that women who had used drugs were probably less concerned about their own health for a number of years and, thus, were less likely (or able) to establish healthier lifestyles in the face of HIV/AIDS. In addition, this strategy was much more common among women who were diagnosed with HIV seven or more years prior to the study (80 percent). As previously noted, women who have been living with their illness for long periods of time may feel a great urgency to engage in a number of strategies to forestall deterioration or onset of AIDS. These women may view healthy living as a relatively simple way to maintain their physical well-being.

Again, for many of these women, particularly those with drug-use histories, health maintenance has not been a priority. For the most part, they were much more concerned with feeding and clothing their children with very few resources than they were about the deleterious effects of substance use on their health. When asked about how she deals with HIV infection, for example, Michelle highlighted a healthy diet and abstaining from drugs:

> Well, I just try to eat better. I'm a real junkaholic so I just try to eat pretty healthy and I wanna quit smokin'. I know that's like the worst thing for me. And, of course, my main concern is quitting the drugs and staying clean, you know? That'll keep me healthy, and actually the methadone is not healthy for me so that's why I wanna get off the methadone too 'cause it's not good for your liver.

As noted, many of these women must cope with their drug addictions as well as HIV. The two conditions can seldom be separated. Successful detox progress often helped them deal with their illness. Michelle explained that her view of self has greatly improved despite HIV. In fact, HIV was an impetus to stay clean. As a clean person with HIV infection, Michelle is able to lead a normal, productive life:

> At least I'm not out shootin' dope. I'm back in college, I'm workin', I'm doin' volunteer work, I'm still goin' to counselin', I got some kinda life, you know what I mean? I got some kind of seminormal life other than goin' to get my methadone every day. Everything else is pretty normal except for goin' to the clinic. And if that's the sacrifice I gotta make, all right.

Some women recalled that when they were first diagnosed they wanted to continue, or return to, drugs. They believed that the virus would end their life prematurely, so why not "numb the pain." The fact that they are living with HIV/AIDS longer than they had originally expected has caused them to reevaluate their thinking and take better care of themselves so they can live as long and healthy as possible. Many, such as Robyn, had psychologically prepared themselves for death, but eventually realized that they needed to concentrate on living:

> I only had two years, something like that, and that was seven years ago. So after a while I kind of—I think I was beginning to get impatient. Like when is this thing going to wind down because I'm tired of all this—insurance paperwork and all these pills, my God! It became pretty apparent that it really wasn't gonna go that way, so the last five years I put more effort into taking really good care of myself.

Similarly, Donna explained:

> I wouldn't wish [HIV/AIDS] on my worst enemy, you know, to go through something like this . . . I know some girlfriends of mine say, "Well, what the hell, I might as well go around and get high." You know, instead of saying, "Well, this is the time to take care of myself, maybe I can live another day longer than I would live."

HIV infection prompted Donna to take better care of herself: "[HIV infection] kinda built me 'cause I know I take better care of myself."

Antiviral drug therapy is central to treating HIV infection and forestalling disease progression. A few women noted that the medication is the most difficult part of their health maintenance regimens. Protease inhibitor regimens or drug "cocktails" are demanding and necessitate planning and strict adherence. As Alicia explained:

> I gotta take the pills every day. That's the thing that bothered me. . . . I take like eighteen pills a day. I try to take them as close as possible as I can. Like in the morning—I go to take them in the morning and I don't eat in the morning, but now I gotta have something, like a cracker or a piece a toast to take the pill. And make sure you don't put no butter on that toast, because if you put butter on that toast the fat's gonna [dilute its potency].

Robyn said:

> I get up at 6:00 am and take my pills. Some of them, they're kind
> of interspersed throughout the day. But the first thing I do is
> make sure I have taken what I'm supposed to take and then take
> everything else I need to take during the day so I can get it in my
> pill container to go to work that day.

Short of a cure, people with HIV/AIDS can strive to maintain their
health as much as possible and perhaps abate, even if in very small
measure, future pain and decline. Although inconclusive, there is evidence that nonchemical health promotion activities may help to slow
disease progression and to alleviate symptoms. Eating nutritious
foods and getting proper rest and exercise may also help to mitigate
fatigue, for example (Douglas and Pinsky 1996). Exercise may also
be linked to improved psychological and immunological states.

It was extremely difficult for many of the women in this sample to
alter their health and lifestyle behavior. Women who were using
drugs and living in poverty had a long history of unhealthy habits that
could not be easily changed despite encouragement from health professionals. Even women who were knowledgeable about what they
should be doing to protect their compromised health found it difficult
to exercise on a daily basis. Furthermore, changing sexual behavior
or condom use were rarely mentioned by women as ways to lead
more positive, healthy lives. In fact, of the women who had been sexually involved since their diagnosis, fifteen (41 percent) reported always practicing safe sex, while eighteen (49 percent) said that they
had never, or had not consistently, practiced safe sex. These women
abstained from condom use because either they, and more typically
their partners, underestimated the seriousness of HIV transmission
or, since both partners were HIV positive, they did not see any harm
in having unprotected sex, despite the fact that they may have been
infecting their partners with different strains of the disease.

AVOIDANCE

Avoidance strategies refer to the ways in which the women in this
study sought to submerge conscious thoughts about HIV/AIDS.

Women who denied having HIV generally avoided thinking and talking about it. When they did have to discuss HIV they generally minimized its seriousness. Approximately 20 percent of the women interviewed tried to avoid or downplay their HIV-positive status. Length of time since diagnosis appears to be an important factor in determining which women choose this style of coping. That is, women who were diagnosed less than seven years prior to the study were more than likely to deny their illness than women who were diagnosed more seven years prior (70 percent and 30 percent, respectively). The relative novelty of their diagnosis may have made it easier for these women to deny their illness. For women who had been living with HIV for many years, however, avoidance may have been a less practical coping mechanism (e.g., these women may have had bouts of sickness they could not ignore). Also, their greater participation in support groups and similar projects may foster a greater awareness of their illness and discourage the use of avoidance strategies. Women who did not have a partner were more likely to engage in avoidance (60 percent). Perhaps women who are not involved in an intimate relationship can more easily deny their illness because they do not have to discuss their status. In addition, situations that act as reminders of one's serostatus, such as sexual intimacy, occur less frequently. Avoidance as a form of coping was also more common among women with histories of intravenous drug use (60 percent). It is possible that many of these women had engaged in avoidance at earlier points in their lives when they sought to legitimate their drug use; thus, this strategy was a familiar way for them to cope with HIV/AIDS.

Women who denied their illness were similar to Jocelyn who is "pretending" not to have HIV infection: "And now I'm trying to deal with that, and I'm just pretending I ain't got it, you know?" When asked if it is difficult for her to pretend that she does not have HIV infection, she says, "Yeah, it's hard. And I don't know how long I'm gonna live. I hope I live to—I'll be forty-five in September. I'm hoping to live to see fifty or sixty."

Women in this category echo Denise's sentiment: "But I deal with it okay. I just don't think about it." When asked who she thought would care for her if she became sick, and if she had given any thought to who would be the guardian(s) of her children, Marie said that she does not "think about none of that stuff." Marie does not feel that she has to worry about such matters because she believes that she has a less serious strain of HIV and is not going to become ill:

> Because I don't know what kind of HIV status I got, but I don't think it's really bad. I'm not goin' anywhere no time soon, I'm not; I know I'm not. I have to believe this. I have to say this to myself, and I believe it's helped me a lot.

Even women who are fairly knowledgeable about HIV/AIDS reported trying not to think about their illness as their way of coping. As Alicia explained, consciously thinking about her health may erode her positive sense of self:

> And I don't even think about it, I just get up and it's a routine, you know, it's like taking my vitamins. That's what I say, "Alicia, just take your pills and get up and go." Because if I dwell on it and I think about it all the time, forget it, I'm gonna lose self-esteem. Everything's gonna go, you know what I mean? And I think of my kids too. I got to take care of my kids, so I can't go nowhere.

There are times, however, particularly when she takes her medication, that reality sets in and she thinks, "Wow, Alicia, you are HIV positive."

Treatment and medical appointments make it difficult to ignore or deny one's illness. In an attempt to "forget about" HIV/AIDS, Laurie does not see her physician as regularly as she should. She reported that, "I haven't been to the doctor in awhile. I haven't been to the doctor because I don't wanna hear it. The less I know, the better I like it."

A couple of respondents avoided their illness to the extent that they evaded the topic when interviewed. Shirley provides a case in point. She was diagnosed with HIV six years prior to the study. She has never married and has no children. Shirley lives with, and cares for, her ill father. She does not have many friends and does not leave home very often. Shirley barely wanted to talk about HIV during the interview, despite the fact that she knew it would be the primary topic of conversation. Questions about living with HIV and her health were often skirted as she pursued other issues, such as her father's health, her aunt's career as a nurse, and other health problems (e.g., high blood pressure).

It is not uncommon for newly diagnosed women to isolate themselves from their loved ones and delay participation in medical care or support groups (Jenkins and Coons 1996). Engaging in avoidance strategies often necessitates social withdrawal. This strategy is especially common among women who are active or inactive drug users. These women often lack knowledge of the disease and the availability of social support, which made them particularly vulnerable to illness and transmission of the virus as well as isolation.

LEGITIMATION AND SENSE OF SELF

Overall, women's coping strategies (except for avoidance) demonstrate legitimation—incorporating HIV into their biographies and maintaining or creating positive identities (Bury 1991). If, as Siegel and Krauss (1991) contend, improving or maintaining self-esteem is a measure of successful legitimating, then these women have been fairly successful. Most of the women in this sample (68 percent) reported an improved sense of self since being diagnosed. As is evident in the excerpts in this chapter, most of these women, although still dealing with the adverse effects of their illness, are striving to find a legitimate place for HIV infection in their lives. As discussed in Chapter 2, the stigma surrounding HIV/AIDS fostered feelings of worthlessness and shame and, hence, disruption. For the most part, their ways of coping have helped them to normalize their lives and, in doing so, led them to maintain or establish a more valued sense of self (e.g., as individuals who can make a difference in the lives of other people with HIV/AIDS).

These women's strategies have altered their social worlds, which, in turn, have helped them to create new selves (Charmaz 1991; Kutner 1987). They have positively reframed a negative situation, suggesting that "people with serious illnesses such as AIDS adjust their expectations of life and, as a result, may view their quality of life somewhat positively," experiencing "meaningful new dimensions of life" despite serious illness (Friedland, Renwick, and McColl 1996:27). Indeed, finding purpose and perceiving themselves as socially desirable individuals, these women were empowered as a result of responding to their illness. Many of their stories reflect a transcendence of self (Charmaz 1987) as these women came to see themselves beyond their physical, HIV-positive beings. They began to value their positive attributes, such as their inner strength and ability to help others. Transcendence also allows for individuals to incorporate broader perspectives into their biographies, helping them to construct meaning (Coward 1994). As part of this process, former assessments of HIV/AIDS are replaced, or more commonly supplemented, with new, more promising interpretations of their illness and lives. As women transformed themselves from drug users, absent or inadequate mothers, and socially isolated individuals to drug-free, involved parents and socially active people, their devalued selves became more worthwhile. Women's assessment of HIV infection as an opportunity for self-growth and social engagement are clearly due, in large part, to their difficult histories. Drug users, for example, were seldom active participants in their own lives; now they are taking action to gain control and purpose (Weitz 1991).

Reconstructing identity, however, is an ongoing and laborious process (Charmaz 1987). One must experience many successes before transcending negative feelings and self-images to emerge with a more positive sense of self. For women with HIV infection, formerly devalued selves may be slowly replaced with esteemed selves. Crises, such as new symptoms or progression to AIDS, however, can threaten women's repair work, rupture newly formed selves, or lead to loss of self. Many of these women have not yet dealt with severe setbacks. It is thus unclear whether their repair strategies will be effective under such conditions. For example, given the physical and emotional commitment necessary to participate in support groups and HIV/AIDS education, it is very likely that women will have to curtail their involvement if they become sick, making these vehicles less effective ways of coping. Friends with HIV/AIDS may be less able to offer one another support as they become sick, and people with HIV/AIDS may have to seek support elsewhere. The homogeneity of the sample referenced in this book and the cross-sectional nature of this study make it impossible to assess women's coping strategies, vis-à-vis their senses of self over time.

Although women's ways of coping have helped them establish or maintain positive identities, they may not be effective strategies for dealing with sickness or HIV/AIDS prevention. Women who avoid or deny their illness, for example, are less likely to comply with treatment. Women who have derived strength from support groups may also unwittingly develop an idealistic view of their ability to fight their illness. Thus, women's coping strategies should be evaluated on two levels: the effect they have on their sense of self and the effect they have on public health issues. Lacking systematic data regarding women's adherence to treatment regimes, this effect cannot be adequately examined, but future investigations should attempt to tease out these inconsistencies.

Women's formal and informal support systems can be instrumental in advancing positive coping strategies and are, in themselves, a coping resource. Familial support, for example, may prove to be an enduring resource for women coping with HIV infection across the illness trajectory. The nature and impact of women's informal support networks are discussed in Chapter 5.

Chapter 5

Social Support:
The Role of Informal Networks
in Women's Lives

Social support includes diverse forms including affective support, practical assistance, and informational support (Green 1993; Lugton 1997; Thoits 1995b). In addition to function (e.g., instrumental or emotional), social support may also be conceptualized in terms of structure (e.g., network size) and perceived quality or subjective assessments of support (Lynch 1998:231). Despite the lack of consistent operationalization, there is general agreement regarding the benefits of social support in coping with stressful events, including illness. The effects of support on morale, adaptive strategies, and even clinical outcomes, such as mortality, are well established, particularly in the gerontological literature (e.g., Berkman and Syme 1979; Ell et al. 1992; House, Landis, and Umberson 1988). Social support may also accelerate recovery from illness and enhance adherence to treatment regimens (Belgrave and Lewis 1994; El-Bassel and Schilling 1994; Singh et al. 1999). Support has also been associated with positive outcomes, such as adjustment to mastectomies among breast cancer patients (Beder 1995), and coping with and managing illness among people with end-stage renal disease (Kutner 1987). As Smith et al. (1985:66) note, "Social support makes patients feel accepted regardless of their condition; acts as a buffer against the intense, negative emotional effects of the disease; and provides enduring interpersonal relations that can be relied on to provide emotional assistance and feedback." Thus, in addition to instrumental help, supportive others may impact how individuals view their illness and themselves, as self-perceptions are couched in social relationships.

Given the importance of informal support in the lives of chronically ill people, it is imperative to gain a deeper understanding of the nature and impact of HIV-positive women's informal networks. In this chapter, the social composition of women's networks is discussed as is to what extent these networks facilitate or mediate biographical disruption and legitimation. In addition, the likelihood of these networks to provide support later in women's illness trajectories is examined.

SOCIAL SUPPORT AND HIV/AIDS

The benefits of social support as previously noted are particularly important for people with HIV/AIDS because of the concomitant stigma and social isolation accompanying the disease (Crystal and Schiller 1993; Herek 1999; Namir et al. 1989; Sontag 1989). As with other illnesses, instrumental assistance and emotional support may be crucial in the lives of people with HIV/AIDS. AIDS is characterized by intermittent periods of sickness and debilitation. Those in the advanced stages of the disease often experience serious opportunistic infections and cognitive impairment that can cause visual problems, ambulatory difficulties, and dementia (Forstein and McDaniel 2001; Morokoff, Mays, and Coons 1997). Depending on the stage of their illness people with HIV/AIDS may require help with activities of daily living (ADLs) such as toileting, bathing, and feeding, and instrumental activities of daily living (IADLs) such as grocery shopping, housekeeping, and transportation. Women may need more assistance than men because they tend to have relatively higher levels of functional impairment and barriers to health care (e.g., transportation difficulties, unstable housing, competing time demands due to caregiving responsibilities) (Crystal and Sambamoorthi 1996). In addition to the more hands-on tasks, caregivers may provide people with HIV/AIDS the emotional support necessary to foster biographical repair.

Further, when faced with a life-threatening illness, individuals strive to find meaning in their lives, gain a sense of control, and restore self-esteem. Significant others may play a key role in these processes by offering emotional support, validating one's experiences, and providing practical help and advice (Adelman 1989; Baker, Sudit, and Litwak 1998; Crystal and Schiller 1993; Folkman, Chesney, and Christopher-Richards 1994).

Despite an extensive literature on social support and illness, relatively less empirical research has been conducted with individuals living with HIV/AIDS, and among infected women in particular. In addition, studies are overwhelmingly quantitative and "the focus upon statistical associations may provide little information about the sociological processes which underlie or generate such associations" (Green 1993:96). Despite these limitations, existing research has identified the influence of social support on various health and quality-of-life measures among persons living with HIV/AIDS. Social support has been found to be positively associated with psychosocial adjustment to HIV disease (Gielen et al. 2001; Grummon et al. 1994; Rodgers 1995), including positive coping styles (Brook et al. 1997; Brook et al. 1999; Lesserman, Perkins, and Evans 1992; Namir et al. 1989), positive self-esteem (Martin and Knox 1997), better quality of life (Swindells et al. 1999), and lower depression scores (Katz et al. 1996; Lyketsos et al. 1996; Meyer, Tapley, and Bazargan 1996; Serovich et al. 2001; Simoni and Cooperman 2000; Vincke and Bolton 1994). Conversely, a lack of social support has been associated with poor compliance to antiretroviral therapy (Catz et al. 2000; Gordillo et al. 1999).

Much of the literature on women and HIV/AIDS, however, focuses on women as caregivers rather than delineating their social support networks. Due to the stigma associated with drug use and gender role expectations that dissuade men from caregiving, women with HIV infection appear often to be abandoned by lovers and family members, and receive less informal support than their gay male counterparts (Green 1993; Kaspar 1989; Rieder and Ruppelt 1988; Weissman and Brown 1996). Contrary to much of the literature regarding social support among people living with HIV infection, men and women in Pedersen and Elklit's (1998) sample perceived that an increase in social support increased over time.

Findings from studies examining the relationship between social support and well-being among women with HIV/AIDS are congruent with those regarding gay men. For example, research suggests that support is a key predictor of quality of life (i.e., daily functioning, symptoms, and anxiety) (Sowell et al. 1997), positive coping (Florence, Lutzen, and Alexius 1994), higher levels of life satisfaction (Heckman et al. 1997), and positive self-esteem (Linn et al. 1993).

The stigma and fear associated with HIV/AIDS, however, may impede support (Conrad 1986; Crystal and Schiller 1993; Wiener 1991). Women with AIDS face considerable stigma and discrimination because they are overrepresented in already marginalized groups, i.e., people of color and IV drug users. Contributing to the stigmatization of AIDS is the fact that it is sexually transmitted, contagious, and life threatening (Conrad 1986; Weitz 1991). As with other stigmatized illnesses, any connection to AIDS is discrediting; thus, those who interact with and/or care for people with the disease may bear a "courtesy stigma" (Goffman 1963:30).

Many women with HIV/AIDS are drug users, or have substance-abuse histories, which greatly contribute to their small and/or tenuous social networks. Drug users with HIV/AIDS may have a difficult time securing support due to their illicit lifestyles and subsequent rejection from disapproving family members and friends. Intravenous drug users are typically portrayed as alienated, isolated persons who lack ties to support networks (Crystal and Schiller 1993; Schneider 1992). There is also evidence that female drug addicts are less likely than their male counterparts to receive parental support, suggesting that drug use is more highly stigmatized among women than it is among men (Shayne and Kaplan 1991). The lack of support these women may receive is especially problematic as the majority are single heads of household with young dependent children—women who may need additional assistance to fulfill this role (Wiener 1991).

Intravenous drug users also appear to rely less on friends for assistance than do gay men with HIV/AIDS (El-Bassel and Schilling 1994; Johnston, Stall, and Smith 1995), although Stowe et al. (1993) found that friends were a more important source of social support than relatives. Their networks may also consist primarily of other drug users, who may be more detrimental than helpful to women's well-being, by continuing the practice of needle sharing, for example (El-Bassel and Schilling 1994; Suh et al. 1997). Informal caregivers to people with HIV/AIDS have expressed concerns ranging from the uncertainty of the disease and effects of stress on their own health to stigmatization and social isolation (Bonuck 1993; Brander and Norton 1993). Although crisis may foster closer ties and increase solidarity, the negative consequences of caregiving may also lead to distancing or abandonment (Crystal and Schiller 1993; Schiller 1993).

Results from Crystal and Schiller's (1993) analysis, however, point to the heterogeneity of this population in terms of familial relations and social support. (However, Crystal and Schiller's sample is primarily comprised of men [77 percent].) Contrary to what might be expected, they found that intravenous drug users were less likely than gay men to live alone and they appeared to have no less access to family support than others with HIV/AIDS. In fact, one-half of the respondents lived with their families of origin and identified family members as their primary helpers, particularly their mothers and other family members.

Similarly, among symptomatic men and women in Crystal and Sambamoorthi's (1996) sample, all respondents reported family members as their primary caregivers. Males generally received assistance from a parent, whereas female respondents were more likely to get help from formal sources or other family members, particularly daughters.

FAMILIAL SUPPORT NETWORKS

Social support was assessed by asking women if they had people in their lives who helped them when they needed assistance (e.g., help with household chores) and/or emotional support (e.g., listening to their concerns and fostering feelings of belonging). Nearly all respondents in this study (95 percent) reported having at least one person on whom they could depend for instrumental assistance, and, more frequently, emotional support. Women's social networks most often involved family members (particularly parents and children) and significant others. Although the role of siblings in providing social support has been noted in other studies (e.g., Bigby 1997; Connidis 1994; Havermans and Eiser 1994; Nichols 1995), including HIV/AIDS research (e.g., Kadushin 1996), many women (67 percent) in this sample did not have close relationships with their siblings, and less than half reported being close to at least one sibling (typically a sister) from whom they received emotional support. Very few women ($n = 5$) identified friends as a dependable support source.

Immediate Kin and Parents

Supportive familial networks were more typical among respondents who did not have intravenous drug-use histories (71 percent). This finding is consistent with some of the literature previously discussed which contends that due to their illicit lifestyles and subsequent rejections, intravenous drug users are less likely to be part of supportive networks. Women with supportive informal networks were also more likely to not have a partner (65 percent versus 35 percent of women who have a significant other). Perhaps women who do not have a partner are more likely to strengthen familial ties, whereas women who do have a partner are more likely to rely on their significant other for support. Women who were diagnosed fewer than seven years prior to the study were also slightly more likely to report receiving familial support than those diagnosed more than seven years prior (53 percent and 47 percent, respectively). This may be indicative of the duration of women's support sources. That is, women's support networks may have eroded to some extent over the years since being diagnosed with HIV infection.

These women were quick to note the love, affection, and motivation their families provided. For example, Alicia said, "If I [need someone to talk to] there's always someone around. I got my family." In fact, some women were surprised to learn that other people with HIV/AIDS experienced rejection and abandonment from their families because the women's own familial reactions to their diagnosis, and relations thereafter, were so positive. As Karen said:

> My whole family accepted it; everyone around me accepts it. All my brothers and sisters, all my friends, all my boyfriends. That's why I could never understand, you know, like someone would say, "Oh, now who else would want you with that?" Everyone I've been with has wanted me with this.

At the start of the interview, Jennifer, when asked to tell a little bit about herself, began by discussing how her family rallied around her when she received her diagnosis:

> My name is Jennifer and I grew up in New York. I'm forty-five. I just moved to the South almost three years ago. Since being diagnosed, I was fortunate I had a very, very supportive family. And all my friends were extremely supportive also. My family got empowered; they read all the literature and educated themselves. Right from the get-go, and this is back in 1987.

In similar fashion, Gina believes that her mother's ability to be emotionally supportive stems from her willingness to become informed, instead of relying on AIDS misconceptions and stereotypes. Indeed, family members who attempted to educate themselves about the virus were more likely to be perceived by the women as important support persons.

Parents, especially mothers, were a key source of support for many women.* Women reported that their parents reacted fairly positively upon disclosing their illness. As with many of the women themselves, parents often panicked initially, then came to be key support persons. Carmen's, followed by Melissa's, description of their mothers' responses are typical examples:

> She started screaming and crying; it was a bad reaction. . . . She was hysterical. I mean, she was screaming, she fainted, she went crazy when she found out. . . . I felt the same way. [I thought] I'm gonna die. But then afterward everything calmed down and we started talkin' and she's been fine with it. She doesn't reject me or anything like that.

> My mother left work. She got sick—she got physically sick, threw up. She didn't know what to do, didn't know what it was, didn't know what to expect . . . so it affected the whole family.

For women such as Denise who did not have a significant other and/or friendship group, their families were their only source of support. Familial closeness clearly helped lessen the blow of HIV. Knowing that they were loved and appreciated helped these women maintain positive senses of self. As Melissa said, "Finding out I had the virus was a shock and everything, but probably because me and my family are closer, there were worse times than that." For some women, HIV was a blessing as it fostered familial closeness. For instance, Marie's relationship with her mother was strained prior to HIV. Smoking cocaine and abusing alcohol, Marie was at times an unfit parent. She described an occasion in which she had failed to pay her gas bill, causing her children to live in an unheated apartment. Upon finding out, Marie's mother reported her to the state child welfare authority. Marie refused to speak to her mother fol-

---

*Sixty-two percent ($n = 23$) either were estranged from their fathers ($n = 12$) or had lost their fathers prior to their diagnosis ($n = 11$). Respondents were less likely to be estranged from their mothers ($n = 3$, 8 percent), although slightly more likely to have lost their mothers ($n = 14$, 38 percent).

lowing this incident and the two were estranged for several months. When her son died of AIDS, however, Marie reestablished ties with her mother:

> When my son died, that's when I got in touch with my mom, and when he died that's when me and my mother really talked about it, that day. . . . And she's like, "You'll be all right; it was his time." She was there—my mother was really there for me then.

Believing Marie would die of AIDs shortly thereafter, she did not cope well with the news and rarely discussed it with Marie. In Marie's opinion, "At first I felt like my mother was scared of it, I could feel it, sense it." It was not until she realized that Marie could live several years without becoming ill or developing AIDS that the two began openly communicating. Furthermore, despite Marie's mother's initial response, she began donating to a local AIDS resource center, which, among other things, provides care to infants infected with HIV. This gesture most moved Marie as it symbolized her mother's acceptance.

Mothers were typical sources of emotional support in this study, but a few also provided instrumental support by helping the women take care of their children and, at times, providing financial assistance, for example. Women who lived with their mothers ($n = 3$) were more apt to reap the benefits of having built-in helping networks. For example, Jessica's mother stood by her despite Jessica's drug addiction and allowed her to move into her home about a year and a half prior to this study: "My mother always welcomed me [home]. She wasn't happy with me, but she always welcomed me, and she always did whatever was necessary to help me get back on my feet. She always has been like that. She's always been there." In describing her mother's reaction to finding out she was HIV positive, Jessica noted that her family offers support without fostering dependence:

> My family has always been very close. I have a close family. . . . They really are supportive. They don't pamper me, but they're there. [They'll say] "Oh, I hope you're feeling all right." You know, that kind of thing, but they don't pamper me, like baby me. But I'm not that type of person who you can baby.

Given the stigma attached to HIV/AIDS and families' disapproval of some of these women's behaviors (e.g., drug use or associating with drug users), disclosing their HIV status was not always an easy thing to do. Despite the women's apprehension about telling their families, they reported feeling great relief when they did. For instance, Michelle dreaded telling her mother that she had HIV infection and waited over a year before doing so. Explaining the secrecy to her mother was difficult, but in the end Michelle is grateful that her mother knows because she is a great source of support:

> She just couldn't understand why I wouldn't tell her, you know, and I just didn't want to . . . Back then there wasn't a lot of information about it. . . . I think it was scarier back then than it is now to tell somebody, you know, and I just couldn't . . . I just had a hard time tellin' my mother 'cause I can just imagine being a mother and having your daughter tell you that she has some terminal illness and that there was no cure. Basically, I just wanted to not have her being all worried about me, and so that's kinda the reason why I didn't tell her. But then I was glad that I did 'cause she was real supportive and she has been ever since.

In fact, although Michelle did not get along well with her mother while growing up, upon dealing with HIV together, she said, "I don't know what [I] would do without her. She's like my best friend now."

Alicia and her six-year-old son are both infected with HIV. Alicia did not want to tell her mother because she is very protective and she, too, feared being treated differently; she feared being discriminated against, despite the fact that she knew her mother "wouldn't throw [her] to the curb or anything like that." Her mother was shocked to see her grandson's picture in the newspaper under headlines reading "something along the lines of 'HIV-infected kids.'" Alicia agreed to have him photographed because she was told "it's gonna be a little picture, it's gonna be in black and white, it's gonna be inside of the paper." Alicia never dreamed anyone would recognize him. When her parents' initial shock and anger subsided, they were more concerned with her health:

> That's the only thing she was mad about because I held it in to myself for like two years. But other than that she was all right, besides calling me for a while, asking, "Did you eat? Did you do this, did that?" . . . And my father was upset because me and my father are tight. But this anxiety came and went and now everybody's all right.

Mothers were especially likely to become overprotective after finding out their daughters had HIV/AIDS. At first taken aback by the news, Julia's mother soon expressed great concern regarding her daughter's health: "She was very—oh God, she was calling me like three times a week, 'Are you okay?' 'How are you feeling?' 'Can I do anything for you?' She was just overly concerned, overprotective." Overprotectiveness, although at times frustrating, was welcomed by these women who knew that many people with HIV/AIDS are rejected by their families. Fussing over them, they noted, was one way that their loved ones expressed their concern.

Spouses and Significant Others

The presence of a significant other, particularly a spouse, is generally associated with perceived social support (Kimberly and Serovich 1996; Primomo, Yates, and Woods 1990). However, research has also demonstrated that there are gender differences in the constellation of helping networks and nature of assistance provided. For example, wives generally provide more care to their impaired spouses than do husbands (Allen 1994). Sick husbands tend to count on their wives for support, whereas wives are more likely to receive assistance from adult children and other relatives as well as their spouse (Antonucci and Akiyama 1987; Arber and Ginn 1991; Johnson 1983; Lynch 1998; Pruchno 1990; Stoller and Cutler 1992; Thoits 1995b; Zarit, Todd, and Zarit 1986).

Women with HIV infection may or may not have partners to assist them and provide emotional support. The presence of a spouse or lover, however, is no guarantee of adequate assistance; support appears to be more closely related to closeness and intimacy rather than availability (Allen, Goldscheider, and Ciambrone 1999). Further, research concerning male caregivers for the elderly suggests that this care is qualitatively different from that provided by female care providers. Male care providers are often unprepared to take on traditionally female caring tasks such as cooking, cleaning, and caring for an ill person (Stone, Cafferata, and Sangl 1987). Rather, men are much more likely to help in instrumental ways, such as providing transportation or managing business affairs. In regard to women with HIV infection, then, male partners may be helpful, but they are perceived as an insufficient source of overall care. This is likely true, particularly in cases where more hands-on caring tasks and assistance with child rearing are needed, which are not part of traditionally masculine gender roles. Thus, male helpers may experience role incongruence between their gendered identities and the caregiving role (Thomas 1968).

As noted previously, women with HIV/AIDS are more likely to have less stable intimate relationships. Further, the presence of support from a husband or lover may well differ according to race, class, and intravenous drug-use history. Although samples of predominantly white and well-educated HIV-positive women who did not have intravenous drug-use histories reported having emotionally supportive husbands (Semple et al. 1993), this is often not the case for marginalized women (e.g., women who are poor, members of a racial minority, and/or drug users).

Among the women studied in this book, of those who were married ($n = 3$) or in monogamous, intimate relationships ($n = 12$) at the time of their interview, most (73 percent) identified their lovers as supportive others who helped them cope with HIV infection. Women with supportive partners were slightly more likely to have had intravenous drug-use histories than those who did not (55 percent). Perhaps these women, many of whom had partners with substance-abuse histories, held fewer requirements for what constitutes a supportive mate and hence were more likely to equate the mere presence of a partner with a supportive other. In addition, women who reported having a supportive significant other were much more likely to have been living with HIV for seven or more years (72 percent versus 25 percent of women who were diagnosed fewer than seven years prior to this study).

The marital context is important. Married women in this sample were most likely to identify their partners as their primary support person who has helped them develop or maintain a positive sense of self. Sheila's husband, Bill, for example, helps her with the household chores and child rearing, but more important, he provides a safe, loving environment that helps give Sheila the will to go on:

> Bill has helped me out a lot, Bill is like my dose of medication. Yes, I'll be honest: it has been Bill. I think by him accepting me that has changed my whole outlook, because now I realize all those things that people try to tell you, that life does go on. I have proved that.

Heather identified her husband, Carl, as her "greatest support person, without question." She said: "We do [a lot together], we're very good friends. He's my best friend. And he feels the same way about me." As with Bill, Carl helps his wife with daily tasks so she can rest after coming home from work. Heather noted that, especially during periods of intense fatigue, Carl has taken on the bulk of the household labor:

> He does more than his share. We've lived in this house—it will be two years, and I don't think I've vacuumed once. He does all the vacuuming. I have to remind myself that I can't take advantage of that. I do what I hope to be my share, do as much as I can. But he certainly picks up the slack, more than his share.

What impressed Heather most about Carl was that he had readily agreed to see a mental health counselor to help her work through some personal issues, including the anxiety surrounding Carl's fear of contracting HIV infection:

> Right now my husband and I are seeing a mental health counselor. And that really helps. We've been going now for two years, every other week. It is a big [time commitment]! We went there because a few years ago my husband kept losing weight—and he's very thin to begin with; he has diabetes. . . . One day he let it come out that he didn't know for sure if he was losing this weight because he had the diabetes or if he could be infected. I didn't realize that that was even one of his fears. And when I heard him say that, I felt mortified and I felt like I have to help him. . . . He was also part of [a large health study] after we first got married—he's very cooperative that way. And very supportive, he's a rock. . . . Then it turned out that the kids were monopolizing every hour. Our relationship was fine, but there were a lot of issues.

Carl not only attends couple counseling sessions, he also has joined a support group for individuals infected with, and affected by, HIV/AIDS. His willingness to learn about the virus and discuss his wife's illness with her assures Heather that he genuinely cares about her and their marriage:

[He has] no qualms about [talking about HIV]. When we go to the support group, I wondered in the beginning: will he be bothered by going to [a group] as opposed to some little office somewhere? And [it] never even bothered him. He's extraordinary! And to put it best, I remember my friend, after she had met him a short time, she described him in one word—selfless. And I appreciate him so much because of what I've been exposed to prior to him. So I just try to remind myself occasionally what a wonderful person I have in my life.

These excerpts show how important acceptance is to these women's legitimation efforts. Acceptance may be especially critical for those who have faced alienation and ostracism due to stigmatized behavior such as drug use. Thus, significant others who have stuck by their mates despite substance-abuse problems, and who accepted the women as they are were seen as supportive. As Michelle said:

I couldn't believe he accepted me with the virus, you know, he's negative. I was afraid to tell him, and he just—he accepted it. He said, "It's fine with me. We'll just be careful." And I told him the things we needed to do if we were gonna be together, and he accepted it. And that was it.

Similarly, Debra's live-in boyfriend and "best friend," Don, surprised her with his loving reaction:

One thing I find poignant [is when] I said, "Sit down, I gotta tell you something." And when I told him, he didn't say, "Oh, I gotta get tested, what about me?" His response was "I can't lose you," and he started to cry. That tells a lot about him and what kind of person he is. . . . Especially for someone that never had that experience, the drug experience, that type of lifestyle, to stick by you. He brought me food in jail and everything. That's how he is. If I do cocaine once a month, he'll start yelling. And he'll say, "Even though I'm yelling, it's only because I love you."

In addition to being a loving partner, Don takes an active role in parenting and shares in household tasks such as laundry, cleaning, and meal preparation: "It's fifty-fifty. Sometimes it's more, he's one hundred percent right now. And I'm in the hospital a lot."

Caring for women's children is an important way in which significant others show support and offer practical assistance. Male companions typically provide short-term care (e.g., baby-sitting) for the children (Baker, Sudit, and Litwak 1998). For example, although Laurie's boyfriend does not help around the house, she believes he is a good role model for her five-year-old son. Preparing for her death, she hopes the two will form a bond that will endure after she is gone:

> He handles him and I basically handle [my daughter], you know, because there's that male/male, female/female [relationship]. My son has a lot of respect for Glen. He needs a male influence, especially since my time is limited, you know what I mean? I've gotta let that connection go, you know, I've gotta let him bond with him.

Generally speaking, however, help with child rearing was much less common among unmarried couples. Women generally shouldered most of the responsibility for child care and household labor.

Many women could not think of specific ways in which their significant others provided assistance. It may be that these women were content to have a husband or lover and, thus, their very presence was enough to help women deal with their illness. In other words, the fact that they had someone in their lives and were not abandoned or alone made them feel desirable and loved. When faced with an illness that undermines one's sexuality and desirability, the presence of a romantic partner offered sexual identity support (Lugton 1997). Relationships that stood the test of HIV offered women reassurance that they were wanted and loved. As Becker (1997:15) explains, individuals "define normalcy in terms of particular cultural images that have salience for them." Because intimate relationships are socially valued, the presence of significant others helped in women's efforts to normalize in the face of uncertainty.

Second, they may not expect their mates to be instrumentally supportive, and thus lacking high expectations they may be satisfied with any amount of attention received. That is, many of these women may have expected that they would be responsible for household chores and child care regardless of their health. Moreover, women whose partners are not the biological fathers of their children may be even less likely to expect great participation from their partners in household tasks.

Children

When to tell their children (if at all) about their illness is extremely stressful as HIV-infected mothers must take into consideration their children's maturity, their ability to accept their mothers' illness and deal with possible stigma, and their ability to keep their mothers' condition a secret (Jenkins and Coons 1996; Moneyham et al. 1996; Simoni et al. 2000). For women with children, telling them of their illness was perhaps the hardest thing they ever had to do. With the exception of Jocelyn, who has not told anyone about her diagnosis, all women in this study with children over age thirteen have disclosed their illness. Women with children under the age of thirteen reported that they plan to tell their children, but felt that they were too young to carry such a heavy burden and/or understand what it means to have HIV/AIDS.

Not surprisingly, for those children who had been informed, their responses centered on fear of losing their mothers, disbelief, and general feelings of grief and despair. There was also a great deal of ambivalence, especially among younger children who either could not fully understand the nature of the problem and/or could not deal with the reality of the situation because the current functional health of their mothers made the illness seem surreal, even unimportant.

Much of the literature on women with HIV/AIDS points to their unique problems, especially the fact that many have to deal with a fatal, uncertain illness while maintaining their roles as primary (and often sole) caregivers for their children (who may also be HIV positive). Clearly, mothering may pose obstacles to living with HIV. For example, women may worry about the future welfare of their children and they may not have enough time to cater to their own needs. Some of the women in this study noted the difficulties of being a mother with HIV infection. For example, Thalia, a single mother of two preadolescent boys, discussed the difficulty of parenting and taking care of herself. When asked if caring for her children eases or compounds the pressures of HIV infection, Thalia replied:

> In some ways [it's harder], because it's like when it's time to take the medication and stuff, I mean I did miss a lot of dosages. But you know, you're out doing this, you're out doing that. They're into soccer, karate, plus working and trying to juggle the work and their activities. You know, just everyday house-

hold stuff, sometimes it does get pretty hectic. . . . But [the children] keep your mind off of it sometimes.

On the other hand, as Thalia implied, women's stressors may also be an important source of strength and support. Women in other studies have also indicated that although concern for their children was stressful, children were a primary source of social support and self-esteem, a reason to abstain from drugs, and a much-needed distraction from HIV-related issues (Andrews, Williams, and Neil 1993). Similarly, Lugton concluded that young children's "demonstrative affection compensated for the attention they demanded" (1997:1190). As with the role of lover, motherhood is an important cultural construct that affords individuals an opportunity to participate in a legitimate social role and hence feel normal. Motherhood may be especially important for marginalized women who have been unable to fully participate in other valued social roles (e.g., spouse, employee). Moreover, mothering may be particularly central in cultures where motherhood enhances a woman's self-esteem, such as in the African-American and Latina communities (Bonuck 1993; Henderson 1992; Lea 1994; O'Sullivan 1992; Quinn 1993; Wells and Jackson 1992). It is not surprising that many women construct their identity in relation to caring. Very early on, girls are socialized to believe that sensitivity, nurturing, and caring are part of what makes them female. Gender roles and expectations that emphasize women's nurturing propensity are then continually reinforced by normative gender expectations as well as social structural arrangements (e.g., division of household labor and inequality in the paid labor force) (Andersen 1993).

Many women noted the strength they derive from mothering, which in turn helps them create or maintain a sense of normalcy. By enabling them to maintain their caring roles, mothering helps them work HIV infection into their biographies, aiding legitimation. Women who did not have intravenous drug-use histories were more likely to highlight their children's role in their repair process (75 percent). It is possible that women's drug use had precluded them from cultivating close relationships with their children and, thus, these ties were less effective in their coping efforts. The length of time they had been living with HIV may also be a factor, although the results are not as marked as drug-use histories. That is, of the women who noted the positive influence of mothering on repair, 59 percent had been living with HIV infection for seven or more years prior to the study while 41 percent had the virus for fewer than seven years. Perhaps having more time to become accustomed to living with HIV/AIDS, these women have since made a concerted effort to strengthen ties with their children. These women were equally likely to have a significant other.

Mothers often referred to their children as great sources of motivation. Carmen, for example, is a single mother raising three children ranging in age from three to eleven. Carmen's children keep her very busy, but she enjoys the time and energy they demand as it helps her normalize her daily life and takes her attention away from her illness. Facetiously, she stated:

> They drive me crazy. I don't have time to sit and think about things, you know? Either they're fighting, or this one is bothering the other one. It's always something, so I don't have— I haven't had really time to [think about my illness].

Sheila explained:

> It's like you have to have something to fight for; my thing was my children. And I'll tell anybody: I think if I didn't have my children I don't know where I'd be. You gotta have something. . . . My kids are my strength, they do help me cope.

Kristen concisely stated what many women expressed about their children and their role in legitimation: "Kids keep you going and give you inspiration, and you watch them grow." Watching them grow is crucial as mothers expressed that they long to see their children become adults and have children of their own. Mothers often did not express specific goals for their children; they were mostly content to be able to still be a part of their children's lives. In Jessica's words:

> They give me the will to stay alive, to keep going. They do. They don't know they're doing that, but they give me a will. Because all I really want is to see what they're gonna become—good or bad. I don't have any control over that. I mean I have an influence over telling them what's right and what's wrong, but I really don't have any control over what they're gonna become.

Raising Shanna by herself, Rachel and her daughter have come to rely on each other. As Shanna gets older, Rachel sees their relationship extending beyond a mother/daughter bond and becoming one of friendship. When asked about the role that Shanna plays in her life, Rachel said:

> Her and her little snide jokes. She's witty; she's funny. She plays it down. She plays a dumb role, like she plays dumb, but she's really not. And when she plays dumb to the point that I'm like, "You don't really believe that?" She'll come out with some crazy remark. So she does help me cope with it, just her sense of humor. She's great, I love her.

Most women who have never had, or no longer have, custody of their children are convinced if they were custodial mothers, they would feel better about themselves, despite HIV/AIDS. Karen lives a very lonely, isolated life. Her five-year-old son lives in the South with her sister and brother-in-law, who have become his adoptive parents. Karen sadly recalled the time she used to spend with her son before her alcoholism shattered their relationship:

> We went to the park, we went to the beach, we went to the amusement park, we went to the movies. I mean, I did things with him, but then at the end what happened was I started drinking heavily and I would just go out to the malls and buy him whatever he wanted . . . [my sister] would baby-sit, and I was going out.

She feels that she would be more active if she had her son with her and she would, in turn, feel much better about herself:

> I don't have my son or anything, there's nothing I really want to do. I mean, if I had my son then I want to go to the amusement park, I wanna head to the beaches like I used to. I mean, this is what I did every year.

Oftentimes, their children's seemingly small gestures are uplifting and reaffirming. For example, Marie lives in a shelter for recovering drug addicts and her mother has custody of her two children. Although she sees them only about three times a week, Marie described the positive effect they have on her self-esteem by complimenting and reassuring her: "My son's always tellin' me that I'm gonna be okay, that I'm pretty. [My children] tell me I don't look sick. . . . Sometimes I'll be sick, like if I had a cold [they say], 'You'll be okay, Ma.' "

Although most women talked about how their children provided emotional support, relatively few reported that they provided instrumental assistance. Children who did provide practical assistance, particularly adult children, typically helped around the house by cleaning their rooms and/or minding their younger siblings. In addition, older children were able to provide transportation to their mothers' medical appointments or social activities. Irene's thirty-year-old daughter, for example, sees that her mother gets out of the house. Irene has been disabled for thirteen years due to asthma and diabetes. At age fifty-four she found out she also had HIV infection. Her poor health, including obesity, transformed a formerly socially active woman into a recluse. Fortunately, her daughter is available to visit with Irene and take her out:

> Oh [my children] are very good. The one that lives [nearby] takes me places and she brings me to her house. She's real good to me. . . . I see her at least two or three times a week, talk to her every day. She lives close by, and if I'm in a sad mood or something she always does something to cheer me up.

PROBLEMATIC SUPPORT

Although most women reported that they had supportive family members, some (approximately 22 percent) described instances of negative support. Negative support is said to come from network members who do not offer assistance to women, who invalidate women's illnesses, and/or who reject women because of their serostatus. In line with this discussion, respondents who had an intravenous drug-use history were much more likely to describe instances of negative support (75 percent). Similarly, women who had been living with HIV for seven or more years were also more likely to identify unsupportive others than those diagnosed fewer than seven years prior to this study (75 percent and 25 percent, respectively). This result is congruent with the finding that women who have been living with HIV for long periods of time are less likely to report having supportive familial networks. Given that these women report less support, it is not surprising that they may be more likely to experience negative support. Women with unsupportive others in their networks were equally likely to have a significant other.

HIV did not change some previously strained relationships. For example, some parents who had distanced themselves from their children long ago because of their children's drug addictions did not grow closer upon learning of their illness. Kelly's mother rejected her years ago, when, suffering from bulimia and depression, she developed a heroin addiction. Kelly hoped that being clean and working to overcome her eating disorder might lead her mother to treat her differently, especially upon finding out she has HIV infection:

> When I went through what I went through, I didn't even see her. She wanted nothing to do with me whatsoever . . . she just couldn't deal with the way I was . . . I didn't find out [I was positive] 'till maybe six months after I got clean and I remember . . . I told [my mother] and I remember how she just looked at me: "What do you expect?" That hurt.

There are times when Kelly feels like talking about her HIV infection and other issues, but, says Kelly, "I haven't had the person to talk about it with."

Some family members further distanced themselves from their loved ones upon learning of their serostatus. For instance, although Rachel was never particularly close to her sister, upon disclosing her diagnosis she has not heard from her again:

> She called, out of the blue, to say she was getting married and that she wanted me to be there. You know, "How could I get married if my sister's not there?" So then I told her about me . . . I said, "Well, it better be a short engagement." And then I told her, and she's like, "Wow." And I wasn't crying or anything. She said, "Gosh, you sound like an ad, a public service announcement on TV." . . . But ever since then she never [called me], you know, nothing. I don't know if it was because she was disgusted by it, taken aback, or what.

Michelle was also shunned by her half sister and, as discussed in Chapter 2, was alienated by her father, whose ignorance led him to fear that his children could be in danger of infection if they were to come into casual contact with their stepsister. Indeed, family members' negative reactions were often attributed to their lack of knowledge about HIV/AIDS. As Dawn said of her mother, "She didn't know anything about it. She was mad. . . . I knew she would react like that. She blamed it on me."

Of women who were married or in a monogamous relationship when they received their diagnoses, few (22 percent) reported receiving an adverse reaction from their lovers or being abandoned. Although many are divorced, the vast majority had separated from their husbands before finding out they had HIV. Upon disclosure, some women were "dumped" or met with cruel responses, such as, "So what?"

Partners who stayed with these women despite their diagnosis were not always supportive, however. Karen's relationship with her fiancé, Joe, best illustrates how the presence of a significant other does not guarantee positive social support. Aside from Karen's sister, who does not live nearby, Karen does not have anyone on whom she can depend for support. Although Joe provides instrumental assistance, he does not provide emotional support. In fact, he contributes to Karen's depression by invalidating her illness:

> He comes home from work and says, "What'd you do, sleep all day now?" Or he'll say to me, "It's all in your head. You know, it's not real." . . . I'm like, "My doctors are wrong? You're a doctor?"

As with Kelly, Karen expressed a desire to talk about her illness with an interested listener, but because her life as a drug addict has precluded friendship ties, she does not have anyone to talk to:

> I have nobody. Like, I don't have any friends now. . . . 'Cause I was on the streets and, you know, people fight for their corners . . . so all I got is him. And if I had to just listen to him raggin' on me all the time—he puts me down all the time. You know, he thinks he's supporting me, but he's not. It's not helping me by telling me, "Oh, the doctors aren't right. They don't know what they're doing. You're just sitting home turning into a drug addict. You're taking too much medication." And I'm always like, "Listen, buddy, you didn't know me before. You don't know what I went through and what I overcame; you don't know nothing—nothing."

Joe also discourages Karen from seeking formal support: "He doesn't want me going to a psychiatrist to talk. But if I talk to him he gets [upset]. It just ends up in a big fight. He doesn't really understand how I feel."

As previously noted, children generally took their mother's news fairly well and offered support, often just by being loving children. Several women (n = 9), however, reported that one or more of their children were unsympathetic, seemingly disinterested, or outright cruel when informed of the serostatus of their mother. Children's reactions early on proved to be a good indicator of eventual support patterns. Some children could muster little sympathy for their mother's situation because they believed that their behavior led to them contracting HIV/AIDS—that they deserved it. For instance, Adele told her young adult children by comparing her illness to that of a basketball star they admire: "And I told my kids, I said, 'You know Magic Johnson?' They say, 'Yeah.' I said, 'Well, you can call me Magic Mom.'" Her son replied, "Well, we reap what we sow." Their lack of concern translates into little, or at best reluctant, practical assistance. Further, her children's actions invalidate her illness. As she explained:

It seems like everybody forgets you're sick. . . . I can't blame them for it. I don't look sick, but you don't get no help. They don't feel sorry, you know? My daughter's been coming over to my house cleanin' the bathroom for me, but I've been giving her ten bucks for doin' it, you know. And would she do it if she wasn't gettin' the money? No.

Similarly, Lisa explained that her sixteen-year-old daughter is often unable to offer support because she does not understand the nature of her mother's illness. Based on Lisa's healthy appearance, Ashley cannot appreciate that her mother is sick and expects her to be able to fulfill her parental responsibilities:

Actually, not too long ago, I said I didn't feel good, or something was wrong. . . . [And she said] "I hate when you say that." She'll tell me she hates if I say I don't feel good. . . . You know, if I say I'm tired she doesn't understand [that] I am tired. I wish she could just have some sympathy, compassion, something, when it comes to that. Because I look good and that's a big thing—that's a real big thing. Well, you look fine, you look healthy. Yeah, but that's not how I feel. If I looked skinny and drawn then everybody would understand. . . . I don't know if I want the sympathy, but I just want her to understand that that's why I can't do [everything]. I'm expected to do everything because I look fine.

Changes in physical appearance due to illness have a dramatic effect on one's self-esteem as well as interpersonal relationships (Register 1989). The absence of such "evidence," however, may also be problematic, as women may have to convince others that they are ill. Indeed, others may base their perceptions less on women's diagnoses and more on how physically healthy or sick they appear to be. As Register noted, "people will measure your health by how you look, extending sympathy when the bags under your eyes turn blue and rewarding your presumed progress when you flesh out and your color returns" (1989:34). Thus, for women seeking confirmation, looking healthy often hinders efforts to validate their illness and secure support. When asked if there are any specific ways in which Lisa wished Ashley would be more supportive, she said:

> Just be more understanding of when I'm tired. If I say I don't feel good, you know, believe me. . . . I kept giving her chances, because a lot of people told me, "Oh, you need to have tough love" and "You need to kick her out." [But] when I die she's going to have such guilt; she's gonna feel so bad. She's gonna wish she had done this and she hadn't done that, and I don't want her to feel that way. So I guess I wish that she would just realize that. . . . She has no respect sometimes for what she says to me, you know? She needs to realize that she's gonna regret that, you know?

Some women continued to provide emotional and practical support to their children, but received little succor in return. When Donna told her teenage children, they appeared unmoved by the fact that their mother had a terminal illness and simply replied, "So what, Ma?" Donna feels badly that they do not take an active interest in her health: "They never said nothin' about it. My daughter never asks me, 'Ma, how you doin'?' Nothin'. She knows I go to a doctor; she knows I take my pills. They don't bother askin' about it." As noted in Chapter 4, Donna helps her children with their household bills and child care, but they rarely reciprocate. As she said, "I'm their support. How can they be mine?" In fact, even when Donna asks her daughter for help, she refuses:

> When I get to the point where I wanna lay [in bed], they say,
> "Oh, Ma, please get outta that bed. What's wrong with you?"
> "I don't feel good today." "Oh, you're just fine, you're just lazy."
> My hip was bothering me one day and I said, "Vanessa, please
> go to the store for me." I can do for that girl, but that girl would
> not move. I said, "What? I can't even pay my bills this week be-
> cause you need food, you need this, you need that." And I said,
> "I got so much on my shoulder I wish you would just release
> me." I'm her support; [my son] don't have no job, I'm his sup-
> port. But I try to help her out because she do feed my son, and
> my grandkids are there. But oh, honey, support I don't get.

Certainly, the fact that their father died of AIDS may account for their reluctance to acknowledge their mother's illness. Rather than deal openly
with their fears, it may be easier for them to deny the fact that their
mother may also die prematurely due to AIDS. In light of this, Donna
makes a conscious effort to discuss death and dying with her children:

> They never talk about death, I have to be the one to bring it up,
> you know, "I'm not gonna live forever. Come on, let me see
> you move. I wanna see what you're doing before I get in the
> grave. I want to know what you're doing." They say, "Yeah,
> Ma." But I think they know, but they think I'm being like a
> mother, pain in the butt. And they ain't gonna give me the sat-
> isfaction; I know 'em, they will not.

Nancy's son was not very demonstrative, but as with Donna, she suspected it bothered her children:

> He's like [his father], you couldn't tell anything [from his reac-
> tion]. But I know it bothered him. I know it did, because since
> then we've talked off and on, and what killed my kids the most
> was their parents were finally gettin' clean and now they were
> gonna die.

In addition to the fear of losing their parents, Nancy's children were
also worried that they may bear a courtesy stigma by being associated
with their HIV-positive mother:

> My kids, especially [my oldest son], still thinks that if I have it
> that reflects on him. That doesn't reflect on him. That has
> nothin' to do with him, and that's what I said.

KEEPING THE SECRET:
UNTAPPED SUPPORT NETWORKS
AND SELF-PROTECTION

With the exception of young children, nearly 20 percent of the women interviewed in this study have decided not to tell some family members about their illness. Anticipating a negative reaction and differential treatment were the main reasons for keeping their diagnoses secret. Only four respondents have kept their diagnosis a secret from their parents, primarily because they felt their parents were too old and frail to deal with the strain of knowing their daughters were terminally ill. As Rachel explained:

> I haven't told them. I couldn't do that; they're in their seventies. Why would I do that? My father's got diabetes and he's on insulin, his health isn't that great. But my mother, she's a rock. She does everything for him. Thank God she's in good health so she can.

Rachel, similar to other respondents, felt that her parents would have experienced undue stress because of the uncertainty characterizing the disease:

> Imagine if I told them now. I've had it for six years. Now if I had told them when I found out and I've been well all these years, oh I would have just added a strain. I would've just helped break my mother's heart, thinking, oh, when is she gonna get sick, when, when, when? How could I do that? And I'm glad I didn't tell them.

In addition to stress, Jessica noted that older relatives were also more likely not to understand the disease and, thus, more likely to be judgmental. Of her elderly aunt and uncle, she said:

> I see no purpose in it. . . . Oh my God, because they're seventy years old. I go swimming in their pool; they'll think everybody that goes swimming in their pool's gonna have AIDS, you know? That's their mentality of this disease; it's not their fault. It's not their fault. Why should they even be updated on it at their age, you know what I'm saying?

A couple of women expressed that their parents and/or other family members would be unsympathetic and blame them for contracting the virus, so to protect themselves, they kept their diagnosis a secret. In Jocelyn's words: "They just are gonna tell me I shoulda been more careful, or 'Why did you let yourself do this?' And that's all they're gonna say." Similarly, Stephanie said of her father and brothers:

> I don't think that they would like reject me or anything, but they would probably be angry and weird, and I just didn't feel like I could deal with certain feelings. You know, because if my father is in denial about my mother's mental illness and my stepmother's mental illness, he's just gonna be in denial about this too. I just didn't feel like I could deal with that. And the same with my two brothers, they're pretty angry too.

Pat, with some encouragement from her mother, also decided not to tell her siblings because she feared it might interfere with her relationship with her nieces and nephews:

> Because I know my sister, the one that's got the two kids, she's finicky. If you have a cold she will not let you in. So I figured that would be the same way, she wouldn't let me see the kids anymore. That's why I didn't tell her.

Jessica worried that if she told the father and guardian of her children he might restrict physical contact between them:

> He overreacts to things. He's a very, he's a nice person, he's understanding, but he's an extremist. He'd be like, "Be careful." I don't want that to be against me, because I can live a normal life. I'm living a normal life and I have been. And I had this for ten years and been around my children all this time and it's like my kids are really up to date on AIDS because they learn it in school, believe it or not.

Jocelyn is the only respondent who has not told anyone about her illness. Living a lie is stressful, but Jocelyn does not plan to tell anyone until she becomes sick:

> I lied to my kids, my whole family. I got ten brothers, nobody don't know yet. They ain't gonna know until it's time for me to

go to the hospital. My kids do not know. . . . My daughters will freak out.

For women to garner support, they had to first inform others of their illness. For those who anticipated negative reactions, though, disclosure was not worth the risk. These women have chosen to keep their diagnosis a secret to protect themselves and/or their loved ones. Women in other studies have expressed concerns regarding rejection, discrimination, verbal harassment, and physical violence (Gielen et al. 1997). Although these fears were realized for a quarter of Gielen's respondents, the rest of the sample reported supportive reactions. Men with HIV/AIDS have also reported receiving more positive responses upon disclosing their diagnosis than they had anticipated (Mansergh, Marks, and Simoni 1995). Although disclosure does not ensure assistance, silence may also be detrimental; nondisclosure may lead to social isolation, increased stress, lack of support and services (Moneyham et al. 1996), and increased feelings of shame (Green 1996).

SOCIAL SUPPORT AND ILLNESS PROGRESSION: SPECULATING ON THE LIKELIHOOD OF FUTURE SUPPORT

Results such as the preceding confirm those of Crystal and Schiller (1993), who contend that the lack of social support for some people with HIV/AIDS may, in part, be based on preconceived notions of social relations among marginalized groups and their informal networks. Indeed, women generally reported that they have supportive others in their lives who help them cope with their illness. By offering positive reactions and reassurances when these women were first diagnosed, their immediate families and lovers helped them combat feelings of loneliness and difference. Similar to the gay men in Carricaburu and Pierret's (1995) study, these women strengthened familial bonds through coping with HIV/AIDS.

Through their relations with their parents, children, and significant others, the respondents in this study were able to participate in identity confirming roles as adult children, mothers, and lovers. However, relatively few women reported having stable sources of instrumental support. Even among those living with potential helpers, many women continued to provide for themselves and help others, despite their health. However, given that the majority of these women are divorced or never married, many do not have a significant other to offer love and companionship, to affirm their sexual identity, or to provide instrumental assistance. Although studies have consistently found that women are more apt to seek out social support than their male counterparts (Thoits 1995b), many women may not have anyone to turn to for support. As noted, stigmatized illnesses may dissolve valuable relationships and/or preclude individuals from forming close ties. Even if women do have potential helpers, they may be incapable or unwilling to provide support, much less intensive personal care. Karen and Joe's relationship illustrates how significant others may contribute to women's stress by being unsupportive and invalidating their illness. Further, as discussed in the previous chapter, significant others, such as Sheila's husband Bill, although enhancing women's self-esteem, may hinder treatment efforts by discouraging adherence to medical regimens, for example.

Emotional support and acceptance are clearly important, particularly in the initial stages of the disease when stigma and perceived difference are more pressing issues than physical debilitation. A fairly healthy group, as was self-reported, the vast majority of these women do not require assistance with ADLs. Over the course of their illness trajectories, however, as they develop debilitating opportunistic infections, the need for instrumental support will arise. In addition, current care practices, such as dehospitalization and outpatient treatment, may lead to increased unmet needs for instrumental assistance among this population (Smith and Rapkin 1995). When the need for care is the greatest, however, social support networks may be less available or willing to provide assistance (Green 1993). For example, among respondents in Namir et al.'s (1989) study, those who perceived health problems as more severe, or reported more physical symptoms, felt that their network was unable to supply the help they needed. Further, lowered instrumental support was associated with more symptoms and lower self-assessments of health (Namir et al. 1989). Thus, whether individuals in one's informal network will be willing and/or able to provide care becomes a paramount concern.

The vast majority of the women in this study (74 percent) reported that they expect those in their informal networks to care for them if they become sick and/or need assistance. Of these, 40 percent nominated their spouse or significant other, 32 percent nominated family members (e.g., aunts, grandmothers, sisters), 28 percent nominated their mothers, and 12 percent nominated their children. However, many of these women's expectations of caregivers may be unrealistic and lead to unstable helping networks. For example, women often nominated potential caregivers who are elderly or geographically distant. Shirley, for instance, nominated her eighty-year-old grandmother and bedridden father: "Oh, no, I'm not worried about that . . . my grandmother is right across the street, and my grandfather, and my father."

Far fewer (26 percent) surveyed women said they expect to receive formal services when they require assistance. A couple of women mentioned hospice care as a probable option. Some women were quick to point out that their families would not be able or willing to be their primary caregivers. As Donna said:

> Oh, nursing-home bound. [My daughter] couldn't even deal with her father for a couple of hours while I go to church. I had to miss a lot of church because he wouldn't pay her no attention. She couldn't stop him from goin' out the door to get hurt, and gettin' on the bus. . . . She has no sympathy, none at all, not for nothin' like this. So I'd have to go directly to a nursing home and sit there. Who am I gonna get? My sister-in-law said, "I'll come up and bring you down my house. It's a long time we known each other; I'll bring you down my house and take care of you." When her brother died she couldn't even come up in the house and thank me for takin' care of her brother, see her own nieces and nephews, see my grandkids!

Living with a significant other was not a guarantee of a future caregiver for a couple of women. For example, although Laurie expects her lover to care for her children when she becomes sick, she does not expect him to care for her. Perhaps naively, she believes that he would make a commitment to her children, despite the fact that he has made it clear he cannot be her full time caregiver. Thus, Laurie has started to consider her formal service options:

> I'd probably have to get somebody because he works and he's not about to give up his job to stay home and care for me. . . . It's just like a mutual understanding, you know what I mean? Like I'm now seriously thinking about getting into the buddy program to get a homemaker in here to help me. Housekeeping

or something, you know, somebody to come in once a week or something and help me with this because it's getting overwhelming.

When asked what the role of a caregiver should be, most women discussed the emotional aspects of support. For example, emphasizing a holistic approach to illness, Marie highlighted the importance of companionship, especially in the later stages:

> To just be there, being company. 'Cause I feel like when people are sick they need some kind of company. I don't think they should be dying alone or sick alone; that makes them sicker. I really think so.

Women stressed the importance of a "good personality," "devotion," and "understanding." A few women mentioned needing help adhering to medication regimens and care coordination, but very few mentioned the more labor intensive, physical tending tasks. As discussed in the next chapter, women with experience providing care to others with HIV/AIDS were more likely to note the multifaceted and laborious nature of caregiving. Hillary, for example, clearly articulated how critical yet emotionally and physically demanding caring is:

> You're everything. You need to be compassionate, and you need to be supportive, you need to be strong, you need to be loving, you need to know how to access different things, you need to know when to ask for help. . . . You have to have a strong stomach so you can clean up, you know, diarrhea and vomit. You need to be able to keep them going emotionally and mentally, and keep them fighting. But you also need to know when to let go, when the time comes and you know that their quality of life is gone and they're ready to go. . . .You have to learn how to let go and say good-bye and you have to learn how to cry on somebody's shoulder and you have to learn how to hide your tears. . . . I don't think anybody realizes how much it takes out of you physically, and mentally, emotionally, especially when you don't have a lot of other people who are willing to fill in.

In general, the women in this sample appeared relatively unconcerned with choosing a potential caregiver(s). Given that most are still in "good" health and have other, more pressing concerns, they have not given much thought to future care needs. Their lack of concern may also demonstrate a deeper, nonverbal sense of denial or an unfounded belief that they will not require long-term caring networks.

Relative to other populations, there is a paucity of research regarding social support networks of women with HIV/AIDS, particularly among impoverished populations (Nyamathi et al. 1996). The results of this study are congruent with others that demonstrate the positive effects of social support on coping with illness, including breast cancer (Beder 1995; Keller 1998), end-stage renal disease (Kutner 1987), coronary artery disease (Anderson, Deshaies, and Jobin 1996), diabetes (Ford, Tilley, and McDonald 1998), and arthritis (Penninx et al. 1997). Indeed, people with chronic pain often seek out supportive others to cope with their illnesses (Schreurs and DeRidder 1997). However, this chapter further demonstrates the unique position of women with HIV/AIDS. For example, relative to other ill populations, women with HIV infection are much more likely to have unstable helping networks. For example, because they are affected at midlife, their children may not be in a position to provide adequate levels of social support, particularly instrumental support.

Clearly, many factors may affect the provision of social support for HIV-positive women, including marital status, socioeconomic status, drug-use history, and stage of HIV disease, just to name a few. Among the women in this sample, for example, those who did not have intravenous drug-use histories were more likely to report having supportive familial networks. Women with intravenous drug-use histories were much more likely to report receiving problematic support. As with other studies, women with intravenous drug-use histories may be especially vulnerable to unmet social support needs. The nature of disease may also affect the adequacy of social support. There is some evidence, for instance, that life-threatening diseases and invalidity foster ambivalent responses from significant others. On the other hand, a poor prognosis may impel others to make a concerted effort to help (DeRidder, Karlein, and Schreurs 1996). Among the respondents in this book, those who were diagnosed fewer than seven years prior to the study were slightly more likely to report receiving support from their family members, indicating that support may wane with time and be scarce when the need for support is the greatest.

Although the majority of women in this study reported that the fatal and stigmatizing nature of HIV/AIDS has not negatively affected support sources, research is needed that examines the correlates of such support. Future investigations that account for the differential impact of sociodemographic factors (e.g., gender and race) and health-related variables (e.g., disease stage and disability) on social support are needed to gain a clearer picture of HIV-positive women's networks and unmet support need. For example, research suggests that women with higher levels of education who have never been incarcerated have more support (El-Bassel and Schilling 1994). Intervention efforts should be targeted at those most vulnerable to ineffective social support systems, such as women with incarceration and active drug-use histories. Further, longitudinal research is needed to monitor women's support over the course of their illness and to understand which ties endure over time, which do not, and why.

As noted, in line with traditional gender expectations, women are often the providers of support and care for infirm family members, despite their own health. The next chapter will examine women's experiences as primary caregivers for their families and will discuss how women's perception of their caregiving role influences disruption and repair. The caregiving experiences of women with HIV/AIDS shed light on their unique position in the AIDS epidemic. Although often not emphasized in scholarly accounts, these experiences help shape their sense of self.

Chapter 6

Women As Carers:
The Dual Challenge of Caregiving
and Living with HIV Infection

Women, despite their own health status, generally feel obligated to care for family members (Barroso 1997a,b; Crystal and Sambamoorthi 1996; Wight, LeBlanc, and Aneshensel 1998). The social construction of gender prescribes caring as natural for women, as part of their innate yearning and skills (Altschuler 1993; Richardson 1989). Thus, societal expectations make it difficult for women to disclose difficulty or dissatisfaction with caregiving (Wilson 1993). Women are expected to support others and be fulfilled by their role, regardless of the self-sacrifice entailed (Lea 1994). Women with HIV infection are no exception to socially constructed gender roles; they, too, are often expected to care for others while simultaneously tending to their own health (Dowling 1995). Juggling multiple responsibilities, including child care and household labor, may interfere with women's self-care, adherence to antiretroviral therapies, and prompt treatment seeking (ACT UP 1990; Flanigan 1995; Stein et al. 2000).

For women who have an infected spouse or lover, the poor health of their partner presents yet another stressor. These women may experience additional anxiety regarding who will care for them in the later stages of their illness (Semple et al. 1993). Because women's domestic responsibilities generally do not diminish in times of illness (Dowling 1995), it is important to examine how caring for others impacts women's experiences with HIV. Thus, this chapter examines how two caring scenarios—mothering and caregiving for infirm adults—affect women's illness experiences, and vice versa. These two scenarios were chosen because of the likelihood of women participating in one or both of these caregiving roles. Also discussed is the likely impact of these arrangements on women further along in their own illness trajectories.

MOTHERING

HIV infection primarily affects women in young adulthood and middle age; periods characterized by participation in multiple roles (e.g., mother, lover, and worker). Given the centrality of mothering in women's lives it is understandable that most women with HIV/AIDS choose to have children (ACT UP 1990; Pivnick 1994; Schneider 1992; Ward 1993). Childbearing symbolizes commitment to a relationship and provides a source of affection, role fulfillment, and status (Bradley-Springer 1994).

Overall, child care was not a major problem for the women in this sample; most women reported that HIV infection did not interfere with mothering. Moreover, with the exception of Rachel, who was initially fearful of infecting her daughter, women were not worried about the possible spread of the virus to their children. In fact, as discussed in Chapter 4, children often helped women cope with their mother's illness. Some adult children, however, were a source of stress as they did not offer their mothers social support and/or invalidated their mother's illness (see Chapter 5). Of custodial mothers of minor children ($n = 10$, 27 percent), half reported having some difficulty with child rearing. Carmen, for example, explained the difficulty of raising her three children by herself:

> In the morning I get up about 6:00. I wake up the kids, get 'em ready for school. I get them breakfast. About 6:30, that's when I start cleaning the house; 7:30 both of them leave. I clean the house, I give [my youngest] breakfast and I put him to watch TV. Then I'll find things to do around the house. If it's not cold, we'll go visit my father until 2:00 p.m. and then I'll come home. The kids are home, and there's fighting: "Do your homework." [They plead], "I wanna go outside." It's hectic sometimes.

Carmen looks forward to the weekends, when the children are with their father and she gets some respite:

> You don't know how I wait for the weekend to come sometimes, just to go out for a little while. And just really resting a lot. Be-

cause during the week I'm with the kids, so mostly when they're not here that's what I do, I sleep. I try to catch up on it as much as I can.

Sometimes Carmen feels overwhelmed and could use some assistance. Striving to maintain this most highly valued social role, chronically ill mothers are often hesitant to seek assistance with domestic tasks (Thorne 1990). Similarly, Carmen is reluctant to ask her parents for help because she does not want them to think that her illness interferes with parenting. Thus, in order to present a capable self, Carmen acts as if she has everything under control, and she masks feelings of role overload:

> I don't tell my family whether I'm having problems or not. I just don't want them to think, "Oh look, she can't handle it anymore." You know, "She seems to be getting worse." I don't want them thinking anything like that. [I want them to know] that I can deal with my kids.

Similarly, priding herself on being a good mother and homemaker, Thalia gets upset when she pushes herself too hard and, consequently, is unable to fulfill her parental responsibilities. She offered an example:

> Last year I was anemic, like real bad, but it was my own fault. It was my own fault, I always think of myself as being normal, and it's like I kept going to the doctors and they're just like, "Are you feeling okay?" "Yeah, I'm fine, I'm fine." But then when my last hemoglobin test came in . . . it was very low, and I was experiencing headaches, I was very dizzy, I was very nauseous, I was extremely tired. I cried 'cause I had to get up and cook the boys dinner. My house was like a wreck; I had no energy to clean it. And if I had to go to work, it took everything I had to do the job.

Indeed, as Thalia explains, part of maintaining normalcy is being able to maintain the role of mother. It is extremely frustrating when women's ill health interferes with their daily activities. Interestingly, Thalia does not hold her illness accountable for her fatigue; rather, she blames herself for allowing her sickness to get the best of her. Struggling to maintain her familial roles, she has come to believe that she should be able to persevere despite HIV infection.

Women working in and outside of the home are more susceptible to role overload and fatigue. These women echo Kristen's contention that being a single parent with HIV infection is difficult because the daily responsibilities do not go away, whether she feels up to them or not: "Life is just difficult in itself, and there's just things that you have to do. Some days you don't feel like doing it and you gotta do 'em anyway."

Adele's children are grown and she is often called on to baby-sit her grandchildren. As her health declined, however, she could not expend the energy that caring for young children demands. As her patience wore thin, she decided she could no longer watch them for extended periods. In fact, with her grandchildren's best interests in mind, Adele explained that when she is stressed, they bear the brunt of her agitation:

> That's another thing, I cut that out. My son was bringin' his [ten-year-old] kid over every weekend. And I said, "No, no more sleepovers, that's it, none of 'em come now." They wanted to sleep over, not just come for a couple of hours . . . First thing in the morning, you know, I got all tired out just gettin' them ready for the day. And it wasn't as bad for me, I don't think, as it was for the kids themselves, 'cause I was bitchy now and tired.

Relatively few women in this sample had perinatally infected their children ($n = 6$, 16 percent). (Five women, 14 percent, became pregnant *after* learning of their serostatus.) Fortunately, fewer ($n = 2$) have lost a child to AIDS. Moreover, three out of the four children born HIV positive now test negative. Reportedly, these children tested positive until they were between the ages of fifteen and twenty-four months. The mothers of HIV-positive children did not report caring for them in unique ways. That is, in general, they did not see their infected children as requiring special attention. These women had a difficult time early on when they learned their children were HIV positive, but are now raising normal, healthy children. For example, Laurie's youngest son tested positive for the first fifteen months of his life. Now, at five years old, Laurie must contend with typical children's behavior such as occasional disobedience and inattentiveness. She recalled the pain and guilt she experienced when she found out her son was infected with HIV:

> Oh, God. Well, what happened was right after he was born—he was about two months old—we ended up having to take him to

the doctor's because he spiked a fever like that! So we ended up taking him to the hospital. And while I was in the hospital his fever kept climbing and climbing and climbing and climbing. . . . They X-rayed him and they found a spot on his lungs; they thought it was pneumonia. The guilt, the guilt—I mean, I actually had to stand there and watch this doctor put an IV in his head. Because the veins weren't big enough, the only one they could find was in the head. Oh, man, it was like, this is unbelievable! The guilt was so bad.

Blaming herself for her son's illness, Laurie returned to cocaine, this time adding new, potentially more harmful drug forms to her repertoire:

And it was like, "What did I do?" Of course that helped my drug [addiction] a little bit more, I couldn't deal with that at all. So he went into foster care and everything. And I was trying, and I was going to the women's day center treatment program. . . . I got in trouble because he couldn't go, so I had no place to put him so I had to stay home with him. But if you miss one day at the women's day center, that's it; they have like zero tolerance. It's like something that you go through every day, but it's like very strong. And it's like you miss one day and it's, "Forget it, we don't want you here no more, you're not serious." That was fine, fine—you wanna kick me out, that's terrific, you know? I'll deal with it on my own. I mean things went on, and I eventually got even worse. . . . My drug was cocaine, and I went from snorting it, to cooking it, to shooting it. And when I got into the needle it was like this is wrong, this is wrong, I've had it. I'm in trouble because I can't stand needles, and I knew if I could put a needle in my own arm myself, that was a problem.

Her substance abuse led her to lose custody of her children and be placed in a strict rehabilitation program. During detox she realized that if she did not make some changes very soon, especially in the face of HIV/AIDS, she would destroy herself and her children:

That scared me, that scared me. I mean, it was like as close to jail as I ever wanted to get. And then I think it gave me like a breathing room because I got away from the drugs. I got clean. I was able to think, you know? It dawned on me: my kids are in foster care. What the hell is wrong with me? Wake up! You know, so what, you got HIV! So what, live for today, give the kids something today. That's what I've been doing.

Maintaining some control over the effects of illness on everyday life is critical to maintaining one's sense of self (Corbin and Strauss 1987). The cultural discourse regarding individualism and, hence, taking personal responsibility for one's health fuels the belief that individuals should strive to control their illness (Becker 1997). As with Thalia, Laurie takes personal responsibility for her troubles and consciously tries not to attribute her problems to her disease. Clean for three years and raising two healthy children at the time of this study, Laurie puts her energy into her home and family. In fact, during her interview, Laurie explained that she loves beautifying her home, proudly displaying all of her decorative belongings because she had been without a haven for so long. The clutter is indicative of all the things that made her house a home, that made her home "normal." For her, the initial horror of having an HIV-positive child has subsided. In fact, aside from normal childhood infections, she rarely worries about her son's health; she firmly believes that he will continue to be disease free.

As another example, Sheila's youngest son was also born HIV positive. She was aware of her serostatus but failed to thoroughly consider what would happen if she became pregnant. Eschewing biomedical treatments, she put her trust in God, and her strong faith got her through her son's illness. As she explained:

What happened [was] I got into this relationship. I was lonely. This guy I met showed me a whole different type of lifestyle. You know how that goes. You move in, you get pregnant, and the next thing happens I'm like, "Oh, my God." And all of a sudden it hits me again, that I'm positive. . . . I go to my doctor and everybody's like panicking, "Oh, no, no, no, you can't have no babies. This is what's gonna happen to you: your baby's gonna die, you're gonna die, one of yous are not gonna make it or maybe both of yous are not gonna make it." And I'm like, "Yeah, right." So they started me out on AZT and I took it for two weeks, and I'm like no one's gonna tell me what side effects my baby's gonna have. I'm not really a pill person. I'm not taking it anymore and I'm just gonna go on faith and see what happens. . . . So they said that the baby was gonna be born with spina bifida. So I had all those tests done, you know, with the fluid and the needles. The baby was born fine, but he was born with pneumonia. [Because] he swallowed some of my fluids. Other than that, you should see him, he's fine. . . . After two years he went on to his own immune system and he's healthy as a rock. That was a rough two years.

Sheila's son then tested negative and she, as does Laurie, now contends with common parenting problems, and dilemmas unrelated to HIV infection. However, initially Sheila was also plagued by guilt:

> There was guilt at first. I'm like, "Why did I do this? I should've listened to the doctors." But then I guess faith—once again it stepped in and said my baby's gonna be fine, just be patient. When I found that he was negative, I was like, thank God for that one.

As these women affirm, they have been very fortunate. Lisa, however, was not lucky enough to have her child's HIV diagnosis disappear. Lisa lost her youngest daughter, Marisa, seven years prior to this study. Lisa's sense of self is largely defined by the pain and guilt associated with her daughter's death. When asked if HIV infection has affected the way she feels about herself, Lisa said:

> Oh yeah, I had a lot of—still do have a lot of guilt [because] I gave it to Marisa. So, I have a lot of guilt . . . If I [had known I was HIV positive] I never, *never* would have gotten pregnant. . . . I have a very strong opinion about women who know they have the virus and willingly get pregnant. I—really, I have a big problem with that. . . . I would never put another child through that, so I never would've gotten pregnant if I had known. I have a lot of guilt—a lot of guilt.

Lisa had no idea that she was infected at the time of her daughter's birth. As a health professional, Lisa now laments that she did not somehow recognize that something was wrong, even though, other than a difficult pregnancy, there were no warning signs:

> You know, I was a nurse. I should have known, you know what I mean? I should have known those signs, I should have. For me,

I had none except during pregnancy. It wasn't a good pregnancy. And I think of this ten years later, and I figured, oh, 'cause my first [pregnancy] was nothing; she was a breeze. I was twenty, so I just figured it was just, you know, [that I was] ten years older, and that was it.

Trying for months to conceive, Lisa and her husband were thrilled when Marisa was born. Upon finding out Marisa was infected with HIV, however, Lisa's husband blamed her and soon the couple separated: "He's got a lot of anger and he must have some kind of blame, you know, for me." Lacking support from her husband, Lisa had to shoulder the responsibility for Marisa by herself. Lisa quit her job so she could take care of her daughter:

In August of '92, when I found out, I resigned. Well, actually, I took a leave of absence, and then I took another leave of absence, extended it. She was really [sick], she didn't come home 'till October. I stayed with her [at the hospital] Monday through Friday. My husband would go up on weekends. And then when we got home she had a central line, G tube, and sixteen hours of nursing, so I stayed to take [care of her]. I resigned. She was just, you know, I didn't want to have to go to work. I have not worked since then. I let my [nursing] license go.

Taking care of healthy children can be difficult. Caring for an unhealthy child as well as other infirm family members while trying to maintain her own health, however, made Lisa's life extremely stressful. Reflecting on her role as caregiver, she said:

It was hard, it was. You know, my daughter's treatment was always in Boston, because locally they don't have a clue [about] pediatrics. So we were up there constantly. Plus my own [care]. I was going several times for my treatments so it was very time consuming. Plus, my mother was sick, and I tried to go over there and help out, make meals and stuff for her. So, yeah, when you're sick and you're trying to be a caregiver, or even like trying to be a parent, it's very stressful; it's very time consuming; it's very tiring. Probably my biggest problem is just having all of this on my shoulders.

PLANNING FOR THE FUTURE: CHILD CARE AND GUARDIANSHIP

By concentrating on the present instead of worrying about when and how HIV/AIDS may disrupt their families, many of these women were able to put off thinking about the welfare of their children. Thus, the women generally explained that caring for their children was not a problem, and they could not see it becoming a problem in the near future. Perhaps even more telling of the women's lack of concern regarding future plans is that, of women with dependent children, only one had made formal arrangements and only a few women had even thought about guardianship plans. Denial concerning the likelihood of decline and death and a lack of potential/suitable guardian(s) were common factors involved in shaping women's planning capacities. A plummeting cell count forced Laurie to consider the future welfare of her children, and she has designated her boyfriend as her children's guardian:

> He's in my will. He's gotta take over guardianship of the kids. I had to [think about it]. Because there was a time when my count went to two hundred, and then it went back up, now it's one hundred and seventy-eight. You know, we're gettin' a little—a little nervous because now it's no longer HIV; now it's AIDS.

A couple of other women have given the matter serious thought, but for one reason or another have not made any formal arrangements. Preparing for her surgery, for example, Debra prepared a statement outlining who she would like to care for her son as well as some of her preferences regarding his education. However, upon surviving the operation, she disposed of the document, reasoning that formal arrangements are indicative of accepting the fact that she may not be alive to see her son grow up:

> The night before I had the surgery done was the only time I wrote something up. [I chose] Don and my mother. I wrote down the schools I think he should go to. I also [named] a couple of [people] who I would like to have some say in his endeavors, in his school, education. [That was] extremely hard. But I figured I had to do it. I tore it up since then, because I came

through the operation. I know that I should, but I can't bring myself [to do it]. 'Cause that's acceptance, and I haven't accepted
[it yet].

Similarly, Rachel has given guardianship preparation some thought
but deems her family unfit to parent, and she does not have any close
friends. Of her family she said:

> She could never be with my family, no way. She wouldn't want
> to anyway. I couldn't do that because she'd either grow up, God
> forbid, an alcoholic or an addict, 'cause they're all like that—ev-
> erybody [on] his side of the family. [And my brother's] a single
> man. He's never been married. How could he? And he works all
> the time. I couldn't do that. My parents are too old. I honestly
> don't know.

Thus, although Rachel recognizes the importance of guardianship
plans, she does not see any viable options. As with the others, Rachel
hopes she will live long enough so that her children will be legally in-
dependent and she will not have to make any decisions regarding
guardianship. Perhaps more troubling is the thought of having someone else raise her child; the thought of being unable to protect her
daughter is extremely unsettling:

> I know that's something I should do, but then one side of me
> says no, I'm planning to stick around, so that's not necessary.
> I'm hoping that I will at least stick around until she gets her own
> place; she wants to move out when she's eighteen. But I just
> hope. Right now I can't say that anybody, nobody, no one's good
> enough to care for my daughter, that's all I can say. No one . . .
> and even though I don't find myself as the best one—the best
> caregiver for her either, I'm trying my damnedest.

Rachel's daughter's anxiety about her mother's death has also pre-
vented her from making formal arrangements.

> She wouldn't even want to discuss it. I had asked her, but I can
> tell it bothered her. [She was] like, "I don't want to hear it; it's
> not gonna happen." But, of course, it would happen. I know
> that's an unfinished thing that I have to deal with.

Working as an outreach worker who is responsible for distributing condoms in poor communities, Alicia is active in AIDS education and prevention efforts. Through her involvement in AIDS organizations and support groups, she is also aware of the importance of making guardianship arrangements. Despite her knowledge, though, Alicia has not been able to bring herself to make formal guardianship plans. As with Debra, Alicia is not ready to accept the fact that she may die prematurely. Psychologically, by not making a formal care plan, she is able to delay dealing with her own mortality and her children's future without a mother:

> I go to a lot of parent meetings down at the health center and they're always talking about it. And I know I gotta do this. And I'm not ready to do it. I ain't going nowhere, you know what I mean? I know I have to do it, but I just don't want to do it now. Maybe if I do it something will sink in, but I'm just not ready to do that now. I'll deal with it when I come to it.

In fact, at one point, Alicia was prepared to go to a nearby meeting organized to inform women about the administrative aspects of the process and to help them make the arrangements, but unable to deal with this issue, she unconsciously blocked the meeting out of her mind:

> They had [a] meeting and I was all psyched up to go. I came home, I made supper, sat down and ate, and I forgot all about it. At a quarter past eight, I said, "Oh shit!" It just blew out of my mind. . . . It was just not meant for me to go. I just can't go do that yet! And I was psyched up to go. I asked my mother if I could put her down for taking my kids. . . . It was all ready for me to go, and I just couldn't go. Something inside of me blocked it out. . . . I mean, I was really upset at myself because I didn't go. Still today, I still can't believe I did that.

Many women had a guardian in mind (typically their parents, followed by their significant other), but have not seen immediate cause to legally appoint them as such. However, most women said they "didn't think about that stuff." Their functional health and an unfaltering hope for a long asymptomatic life made guardianship arrangements seem unnecessary. It is easier for these women to contemplate their own pain and suffering than it is to think of the pain of their children. These women may accept the fact that they have HIV/AIDS, but they are less accepting of the fact that they may be incapacitated or die before their children are mature enough to take care of themselves.

CARING FOR ADULTS WITH HIV/AIDS

For most of these women, parenting was a welcome, if seldom planned, caring arrangement—women wanted and expected to become mothers and raise their children. Caring for infirm adults, on the other hand, was not an anticipated role. However, as with women in general, these women assumed the role of caregiver rather than abandon those in need.

A few women had been primary caregivers to people with AIDS prior to their interviews. For some, caring was a labor of love. For others, caring was a moral obligation. Regardless of what motivated these women to care, the costs and the benefits are clear. Three women, Sheila, Hillary, and Donna, were primary caregivers to their significant others. Although they represent only 8 percent of this sample, these women's stories illustrate a pervasive concern among health care professionals who treat women with HIV/AIDS. That is, having to care for others while dealing with their own illness, women may be overburdened to the extent that their responsibilities negatively affect their own health.

Sheila took care of her first husband. Unlike Sheila's current marriage, her first marriage was "a living hell." As discussed in Chapter 2, Bob was a violent man and Sheila married him because she was pregnant with his child and, at her parents' admonition, she felt morally obligated to do so. When they married, Sheila had no idea that Bob was using intravenous drugs nor did she know that he was infected. Sheila left Bob, still unaware that he was HIV positive. When he caught up with her, however, he had lost a great deal of weight and looked very sick. Bob told Sheila he had cancer, but their test results confirmed that Bob did not have cancer, rather, they both had HIV infection. Despite the abuse and deception, Sheila could not turn her back on Bob. Throughout his illness, and especially during the last six months of his life, she "did everything for him." Soon Bob required around-the-clock assistance, so Sheila had to leave her job to provide full-time care. Despite the way he treated her, Sheila cared for him with respect, sacrificing her time, her energy, and her family's happiness:

> I always did what I had to, to make him comfortable. . . . I gave him my bedroom and I would sleep with my kids. I always thought I was keeping him clean. He couldn't walk or anything. You have to put the [undergarments] and everything on him. He would never wanna eat . . . I'm paying for [his] medical bills, he doesn't have a job, this is on my medical coverage. I am sacrificing my job, my two kid's welfare, and my own to take care of this man who has abused me, beat me.

Perhaps in part due to later-stage dementia, Bob continued to assault Sheila until he died: "He was evil at everybody. I would try to feed him; he would throw food at me. I mean, he would take his feces and just throw 'em. I went through all types of abuse."

Along with the stress of daily tending, Sheila also had to contend with Bob's death. One day as Sheila left to request an extended leave of absence, she had a feeling that would be the last time she would see him alive:

> He died in the house, and that was a weird day. . . . I went in the room, I looked at him, and you could tell. He couldn't talk anymore, he was so small, he was like a skeleton with layer of skin, and he couldn't talk. And I said, "If you could hear me, just nod." And he nodded. I said, "I'll be right back." And I had asked him did he want to go to the hospital, but during all that time we would put him in hospitals and he refused the treatment, he wanted to die at home, so I said okay fine. I felt his body and you could tell it was like icy, getting cold, very, very, very, very cold. So I said, "Look I'm gonna go to my job and I'll be back." And it was weird: I made it to my job. I get back in my car and all of a sudden, this weird feeling just came over me. I knew.

Even though Bob became too ill and frail to hurt Sheila again, the sexual abuse she endured has had a lasting effect on her sense of self and, consequently, the intimacy between her and her current husband, Bill:

> He's startin' to notice. [He'll say] "You don't even like to be touched; you don't even like to have sex anymore." And I'm

like, "I've never been a sexual person." I think because my first husband—I hated him so much because of the things he did to me, and it was more of a rape thing. If you look at the ages between my kids, you know, like nine years apart. And I think . . . the time I conceived my second daughter was actually rape because that's what he did, that's how I conceived her. I just got turned off of sex, and I'm still like that to this day because all those fights and things we used to have, he used to take away my self-esteem. He destroyed that. And I always thought I was ugly.

When asked to speak about the tension between having a connection with this man, yet despising him, Sheila explained that religious and humanitarian morals guided her actions:

There was days where he would like beat me up and take my paycheck, and we had no food or anything. Regardless, he was my husband; he was a human being. I just knew that I just couldn't leave him alone on the street to die like that. And you don't think about what you have to do, you just do it and you think about it later. Now when I go back and I think of those times, I'm like, why did I do it? And I think it was mostly [because] I'm a kind of spiritual person so I believe that God just guided me, you know? . . . I believed that anybody else that he had abused the way [Bob] abused me and my kids wouldn't have did it, they would've left him out in the street. . . . So what I did, I buried him underneath a tree where my natural mother was. I gave him [a proper burial], and people said to me, "Why are you spending this money?" Once again, he was my husband; he was human.

As noted, Hillary's second husband, Charles, also had AIDS. His diagnosis shattered the couple's plans and put their dreams on hold. Charles's failing health was a red flag for Hillary, who knew enough about the virus to associate his intravenous drug-use history with AIDS:

He kept going to [the] doctor, and he kept saying, "Well, it seems like bronchitis." And they kept changing the antibiotics, and none of them worked. And over a period of two months he lost thirty pounds, and I don't know how he kept walking. By 1988 people knew about HIV and AIDS, and I always read a lot, watched the news, and TV, and so I was aware. And in the back of my head I was thinking he's high risk for HIV and AIDS, because he was an IV drug user. But I didn't want to say that to him, unnecessarily. I kept hoping the doctor would pick up on something, but he just didn't. Charles just kept getting worse.

Hillary pleaded with Charles to divulge his drug-use history to his doctor so he would test him for HIV. Shortly thereafter, Charles was diagnosed with AIDS.

Upon rejection by his mother, Charles decided not to disclose his diagnosis to anyone else. Although Hillary understood and respected her husband's wish for secrecy, their isolation left her feeling alone and longing for emotional support:

> He was scared to death to let anyone know after his mom walked away from him when he told her of his disease. She didn't want anything to do with him. He decided he couldn't tell anybody else in his family. And I couldn't get any support down there. Emotional [support], more than anything, is what I needed. I knew my children would understand . . . but we kept it a secret until he passed away.

Hillary tested positive soon thereafter, but caring for Charles allowed her little time to cater to her own emotional and physical needs. Soon she noticed that caregiving was taking a toll on her health:

> I was much sicker for a while. I think it wasn't all HIV. I think a lot of it was the stress of taking care of my husband, 'cause I was his primary caregiver, and emotionally and physically it really wore me down. And so my T-[cell] count went in the toilet and I was having symptoms. I was no longer asymptomatic. I got my full-blown AIDS diagnosis in 1995.

Hillary aptly described the labor of caring as physically and emotionally exhausting. In addition to the physical tending, Hillary was also tending to his psychological well-being, trying to lift Charles's spirits and alleviate the guilt he felt for his dependence on his wife:

> I did a lot for him, and I'm never sorry I did. I had to. In the last three weeks of his life he lost his sight to cytomegalovirus retinitis, he lost his ability to walk, he became incontinent. He

couldn't control his bladder and his bowels. And then he pretty much lost his mind. I had to clean him, and put Depends [undergarments] on him. And he would cry, and he would say to me, "I can't believe my wife is reduced to doing this for me." He always felt guilty. He used to say to me, "It's not enough that I did something and I'm dying from this, but I had to take you with me." And I'd say to him, "You didn't know." But it never was enough to convince him.

In an effort to raise her husband's morale, Hillary often had to conceal her own fears and despair:

> I used to go away when I got upset. I wouldn't let it show. And as soon as I got him so he was comfortable, I'd go sit out on the doorstep and I'd cry and get it out, you know? And I got in therapy so I had some place to go and dump it all, instead of thinking I could hold it all inside.

Caring for Charles was not Hillary's only caregiving experience. Less than a year after Charles died, Hillary met Jim at an AIDS support group meeting. They dated and eventually moved in together. Over the next three years, when Jim became ill, Hillary revisited her role as primary caregiver.

Jim was a recovering alcoholic. As Jim's health deteriorated and he sought the comfort of alcohol, he became verbally abusive. Similar to Sheila, Hillary decided to help Jim despite his addiction and his abusiveness:

> I also physically suffered from that too because of the stress. He got dementia, so it was really hard taking care of him. I mean he didn't have his mind toward the end. . . . As he started to get really sick, and he knew the end was getting there, he couldn't handle it, so he went back to drinking. And when he drank, he was abusive. And it was verbal abuse and I put up with more of it than I should have, but it's difficult enough to leave somebody you have feelings for. When that person is dying, it's really hard to walk out the door. But when it got to the point where he physically abused me once, I left.

When Jim became too ill to inflict physical harm, however, Hillary resumed caring for him:

I went back and I took care of him. I didn't go back into a physical relationship with him. That was one of the agreements, that I would go back to take care of him so he would be able to have somebody with him and he could die in his own place . . . so I went back, I stayed with him, I took him through his death and his dying, and I don't regret it. If I had to do it again, I'd do it again.

Unlike the case with Charles, Jim's family was emotionally supportive, but they did little to alleviate the physical demands of caregiving, leaving Hillary to shoulder all the responsibility: "His family was great to me. And I still have a good relationship with his mom, but she couldn't cope with taking care of him, and [n]either could his sister, so it all fell basically on me." Reflecting on these experiences, Hillary discussed their effect on her health:

I put [my T-cell count] in the toilet twice because of that. And emotionally, I mean toward the end with the second one with the dementia, it was like night and day I was awake, because I slept with one eye open. I went on sheer adrenaline and willpower and that was it. I don't know how much longer I would have been able to do it if he hadn't died when he did. . . . It was a long time, and it did a number on me.

Following Jim's death, Hillary made a conscious effort to take better care of herself and restore her own health by resting and getting enough sleep. Although emotionally and physically taxing, caregiving also allowed for personal growth and fulfillment: "It was great in many ways, having to take a person through their death and dying." However, even with formal help, she doubts she could ever take on the primary caregiver role a third time:

[My husband couldn't] take care of himself at all; he relied on everybody else, mostly me. And it happened with the second man. . . . I still was the one that bathed them most of the time, even though they had a home health aid come in, because both of them didn't really want anyone else doing for them as long as I could. They get real dependent on you, and they get past the embarrassment of you changing them and cleaning them, but they still don't like it when somebody else has to do it. And they'll fight you as long as they can on that, losing their independence, that's hard. . . . And I don't think I can go through that again. . . . I don't even know if I could handle that, to be honest with you, physically, no.

Donna has always cared for others—her children, infirm elders, and the father of her children, Ron. Donna and Ron were together twenty-three years but never married. In many ways, Donna's story closely resembles those of Sheila and Hillary. She noted the distress and sacrifice associated with watching someone you care about go through a painful death: "He just died like two years ago. But I thank God he was taken; he was in a lot— *a lot* of pain. I took care of him the whole time he was sick, and I took two years out of work." When caring for Ron, Donna ignored her own health. In fact, she did not find out she had HIV infection until four years after Ron was diagnosed. As with Sheila and Hillary, Donna was involved with a drug addict, making a "normal," happy relationship an elusive hope. Despite their history, his repentance moved Donna, and she soon forgave him:

> When he got sick he was real bad off, couldn't get out of bed and stuff. Before his mind had lost, he said, "I'm really sorry for what I did to you." And "Please take care of my children." And "Thank you for what you're doing for me." I—see, I'm about to cry. Oh, that just took it out of me. So I didn't blame him, you know?

More than the others, Donna emphasized the gratification she received from caregiving:

> [I did] a lot of hands-on care. I did intravenous. I did everything for that guy. It was like a nurses' aide position, you know, with a little treatment involved. Yeah, but I enjoyed it, I really did.

Whereas the other women could not imagine reliving these experiences, Donna would not think twice about caring for someone in need. She also believes that it would be less stressful to care for someone other than Ron:

> I love it. Stressed me out because it was him; if it was somebody else I wouldn't get stressed out. I love takin' care of people that need it. . . . I love doin' it because, you know, I enjoy the feeling of nursing all the way around.

THE CONSEQUENCES OF CARING

Scholars, particularly in the field of gerontology, have done a great deal to draw attention to women's caring labor for the chronically ill (e.g., Abel 1990; Alford-Cooper 1993; Barusch and Spaid 1989; Brody 1981; Graham 1983; Stoller and Cutler 1992). The voluminous literature on caregiving has identified the sociodemographic trends in caregiving and the social implications of women's caregiving (Schiller 1993). Concepts such as "women in the middle" and "caregiver burden" have helped draw attention to the unique stressors caregivers face when lacking social and structural supports (Brody 1981; Schiller 1993; Young and Kahana 1989).

Similarly, HIV/AIDS researchers have highlighted women's invisibility in the AIDS epidemic, especially as caregivers to other people with AIDS. The unpaid labor of female carers has been supported by gender ideologies that reinforce women's roles as nurturers (Lea 1994). Also, as with the gerontological research, this growing literature notes how women are faced with multiple demands that heighten the burden of caring. Clearly, then, there are many similarities between HIV-positive women and other female caregivers. However, the social place of women with HIV coupled with (and related to) the invisibility of women's work intensifies the precarious position of HIV-positive caregivers. Unlike other caregivers, HIV-positive caregivers are more likely to be women of color and/or women of lower socioeconomic classes. Thus, in addition to the strains of caregiving, these women must contend with environmental stressors such as poverty and inadequate housing, which undoubtedly contribute to their already compromised health (Schiller 1993; Wyche 1998). In addition, they may be providing care to the people who infected them—or, even worse, who infected them and kept their HIV-positive status a secret.

For the women in this sample, HIV has not posed great obstacles to parenting. Although some women have experienced HIV-related and nonrelated difficulties, in general, they do not consider parenting to be a contributing factor to the disruption caused by HIV/AIDS. Hopeful that their medication cocktails will forestall sickness and decline, these women are not overconcerned about an increasingly common phenomenon: HIV-positive women neglecting their own health care needs to provide care to other people with HIV/AIDS.

Whether optimistic or naive, these women viewed mothering as a positive experience that helps them cope, rather than a burden that may compromise their own well-being. Even women who did not have custody of their children were proud of their roles as mothers. Indeed, women constructed their own meanings of caring—conceptions that differ from the more typical definitions of caregiving but nonetheless reaffirm women's nurturing role.

Overall, for these women their continuation of caring mitigated the disruption caused by HIV infection. The stability of their caring roles offered continuity and allowed women to incorporate HIV infection into their lives or accomplish legitimation. In other words, being able (to some extent, at least) to manage home and family life provided women with some control in the face of an uncertain, incurable illness. Similarly, as in Marie's case, involuntary relinquishing of caring responsibilities makes integration of the illness and restoration of identity more difficult.

As noted in Chapter 5, individuals make sense of their lives, which include health and illness, in terms of cultural discourses. Cultural discourses become moral discourses as they dictate how we are to live our lives (Becker 1997). As such, the cultural discourse regarding womanhood teaches women that their role as women is largely tied to their ability to nurture and protect others (Gilligan 1982). Mothering, in turn, allows these women to see themselves as worthy, normal women who, despite failing in other realms, have a claim to social acceptance and status (Becker 1997). Further, it is possible that for some women, being a good caregiver allows them to seek social and/ or religious absolution for their own illness.

Although less common among the women in this sample, caring for other people with HIV/AIDS proved to be a double-edged sword. As with caregivers in other studies, women generally felt morally obligated to care for others (Brander and Norton 1993; Songwathana 2001), and these women did all they could to maintain their relationship with their loved ones and help them through their illness (Bunting 2001; Linsk and Poindexter 2001). On one hand, caregiving drained them physically and emotionally. Caring required all the energy they could muster, and in some cases, as noted, the women helped men who were responsible for their pain, anguish, and even their illness. Not surprisingly, these women noted the negative consequences of caregiving, including strained resources, loss of employment, social isolation, and psychological and physical fatigue (Bonuck 1993; Brander and Norton 1993). These consequences are not unique to AIDS caregiving (Thompson and Pitts 1992) but, as already discussed, these consequences may be more problematic due to the stigmatized, uncertain nature of the disease.

On the other hand, caregiving helped these women see themselves as decent, selfless people. The identity-building nature of caregiving clearly comes through in these women's narratives. The personal integrity and strength the women derived from caring often compensated for the sacrifices they had to make. Because of these women, men who may have otherwise died alone were able to live the remaining days of their lives in a caring, supportive environment. They may have been lacking skills and resources, but it was because of the women that other human beings died with dignity.

Will these women be able to continue to fulfill their parental responsibilities in the later stages of their illness? What will happen if they become sick and are called upon to care for others? These questions are important due to the likelihood that they will become impaired while their children are still dependent on them for personal effects and emotional nurturance. It is also not unlikely that these women will again be caregivers to infirm adults at some point in their lives. For example, traveling in social circles populated by other people with HIV/AIDS, women, such as Hillary, some women may meet HIV-positive mates who may become ill. In addition, as noted, of those who are sexually active, slightly less than half (46 percent) were not practicing safe sex. Their lovers, then, could become infected and eventually need assistance. Because it is less common for women to abandon their loved ones in times of illness, they may well take on this caregiving role despite their own needs. In order to avoid feelings of inadequacy and maintain their senses of self, women may deny or downplay their own sickness to persevere in their role as caregivers. Ignoring the symptoms of infection, these women further threaten their already fragile immune systems. Furthermore, formal agencies, in line with traditional gender roles and women's greater capacity to care, may offer less assistance to women in obtaining additional help than to their male counterparts (Karon 1991; Wright 1983).

This chapter examined an important scenario, one which impacts living with HIV/AIDS. In similar fashion, the next chapter presents an analysis of the place of HIV/AIDS in women's biographies relative to other assaults on the self. Chapter 7 demonstrates how women reconstruct the meanings they initially attached to their illness, leading most to conclude that HIV/AIDS is not the most disruptive life event they have experienced.

Chapter 7

Multiple Assaults on Self:
The Relative Impact of HIV/AIDS
on Women's Lives

The growing literature regarding women and the AIDS pandemic is broadening our knowledge of the unique social situation of women with HIV/AIDS. These women, mostly poor women of color, must deal with multiple problems, including poverty, violence, and limited access to health care. For women who are IV drug users, their addiction compounds these problems. Intravenous drug users, for example, are often ostracized from their families and lack a positive social support network (Schneider 1992; Shayne and Kaplan 1991). The majority of female drug users are single heads of household with young dependent children who have "historically . . . been tangled in a web of poverty, illness and oppression; by the dictates of racism and poverty, they are disempowered, disenfranchised, and alienated from traditional sources of help and support" (Wiener 1991:377).

Given that these women typically face multiple assaults on self, what meanings do they attach, in retrospect, to HIV/AIDS? Is having a life-threatening illness considered the most disruptive life event? What differentiates respondents for whom HIV is most disruptive from those for whom it is not? This chapter addresses these questions and explains how women narratively reconstruct the meaning and significance of HIV infection in light of other disruptions. It is important to note that the majority of respondents have lived relatively symptom free since the time of diagnosis. Thus, their initial fears and expectations regarding the progression of their illness have not been realized for the most part. Most reported having few HIV-related symptoms. Perhaps more important, most reported good functional health, i.e., none reported difficulty with activities of daily living and very few have trouble with instrumental activities of daily living.

Therefore, even if they do have some health problems, these have not greatly interfered with their daily living. These two aspects—being asymptomatic and functionally well—are central to how women reconstruct the meanings attached to HIV infection and its consequences for everyday life.

"I'M USED TO BEING ATE UP ANYWAY"

Despite the fact that HIV infection posed an immediate threat to women's sense of self and has had a lasting impact on their future plans and goals, in hindsight many women did not consider HIV to be the most disruptive event in their lives. At the time of their interviews respondents had been living with HIV infection for an average of six years, giving them time to integrate their illness into their biographies. During the interviews women were asked to talk about the difficult times in their lives, how these events affected them, and how they have dealt or are dealing with them. As they recounted their lives and the disruptive events they have experienced, over half (65 percent, $n = 24$) revealed that other disruptive events were, in retrospect, more consequential than HIV infection. Involvement in abusive relationships, being separated from their children, and substance abuse were deemed more disruptive than HIV/AIDS.

Violence

The social situations (e.g., poverty, substance use, economic dependence, and sex-for-drugs exchanges) of many women with HIV/AIDS have exposed them to violence and abuse (Monti-Catania 1997; Smith et al. 1996; Zierler 1997; Zierler et al. 2000). Violence was a common experience for women in this sample—33 percent have been involved in abusive relationships at some point in their lives; 14 percent have been abused by one of their parents or another family member; and 8 percent reported other incidents of violence, most often when they were involved in prostitution.

For some, such as Sheila, who had undergone long-term intimate violence, these violent periods were the difficult times that crushed their self-esteem. Sheila is now happily married to a supportive, loving man. However, her first marriage was a living hell. Sheila's first husband "destroyed [her], he took everything from [her]." Describing her relationship relative to HIV, Sheila said:

> I would say the hardest time was the abuse . . . because when you're in an abusive relationship, your body's just dead. It's just like a robot that's doing what it has to do. Compared to just living with HIV, I'd rather live with having AIDS and HIV any day compared to being abused. . . . When you're abused you have nothing, I had *nothing*. I had no feelings, I had nothing. I was just one cold person.

Becky, who has AIDS, described how living in an abusive relationship affected her:

> I was totally controlled by fear, totally. I mean, we would fight verbally over my kids, but he would totally do what I would say to the contrary. He would go back in their room or something and say something to them that I totally didn't agree with. And then he'd come back and say, "If you say one fuckin' word . . ." He used to get so paranoid when we would go out, very sick, if somebody would even look at me. One time he told me that he was gonna burn my eyes out because he said, "They're always looking at your eyes and you're looking at their eyes." And he would take it out on me and say, "You're already probably in bed with him." It was very, very sick.

Becky had to "escape" the relationship by moving from the South to the Northeast to live with her mother because "every time [she] told him [she] was gonna leave he'd either absolutely bawl like a baby or he'd get violent." In comparing the abuse to having HIV infection, Becky said, "Oh, my God, nothing compares to abuse."

Similarly, in referring to HIV infection, Geraldine said, "This is a piece of cake [compared to] living with an abusive person." She elaborated on the constant fear accompanying abuse:

> If you're living with somebody who's like psychotic and dangerous and is a threat to your life, you don't know what to expect. You don't know if you're gonna wake up in the morning, you know what I mean? And you don't know if you're gonna be maimed. . . . I had a husband who had a crossbow with razor-tipped arrows and was jealous, and accused me of fooling

around all the time. He used to feel the hood of my car when he came home from work, to see if I just snuck in before him. I mean, would you fool around on a guy like this? He held a sawed-off shotgun to my head. This is scary. Someone telling you, you got a disease that's gonna kill you. Yeah, all right. You know? I'm lucky I'm still here, so there's no comparison, you know?

Donna, too, has long dealt with drug addiction, abuse, and poverty. She struggles to make ends meet in addition to financially helping her two adult children. Donna emphasized that even when she and her longtime boyfriend were using drugs, she always made sure that her salary went to feeding and clothing her children. In large part because of her strong religious faith, Donna has an amazingly positive attitude despite the burdens she bears. Her children are not very supportive nor do they help her instrumentally or financially. In fact, she continues to take care of them. She worries about her children's futures: Will they be able to abstain from drugs? Will they be able to care for their own children? Will they be able to survive economically without her? These questions overshadow concerns about her own health and welfare. As she explained that the strain of taking care of her family is more profound than HIV, she questioned how these stressors could be more troubling than a fatal virus. She has not come up with an answer to this question, but she knows that, for whatever reason, they are more distressing:

> I think it's easier to deal with the HIV than the stress in my life. I don't know what it was, if stress really could be worse than HIV, but I think it was, to me. I worry about bills. I worry about my daughter, my son. If my grandkids are being proper, 'cause my daughter is really mean. I mean she's strict, a little bit over strict.

Mother/Child Separation

It is not uncommon for women with HIV infection to lose custody of their children (Pivnick et al. 1991; Smith et al. 1996). Estimates from several studies of HIV-infected children show that less than 50 percent are living with their mothers due to substance abuse during pregnancy, maternal illness, or death (Mellins et al. 1996). Incarceration, participation in drug treatment programs, poverty, and/or removal of children by child-welfare authorities are typical scenarios of mother/child separation (Pivnick et al. 1991). Similarly, many of the women in this study had to contend with giving up custody of their children, either voluntarily or involuntarily. At the time of the interviews, seven women with children under age eighteen were non-custodial mothers, whereas nine women had custody of their children. Two respondents had custody of their children at the time of interview but had been temporarily separated from their children in the past. For some women, the separation was a voluntary decision. For instance, some women relinquished custody of their children to their mothers and sisters because they wanted the best for their children and knew that in their current situation they could not provide that. Others were forcibly separated from their children because of their alleged incapacity to provide proper care for them, most often because of substance abuse.

Some of these women explained that being separated from their children was a severely disruptive event that forced them to relinquish a role that gave a sense of purpose and continuity to their lives. Marie, for example, is a thirty-one-year-old African-American woman who had been living with HIV infection for six years and had been living apart from her children for two years at the time of the interview. She said, "When I gave my mom my kids, that really hurt me a lot. I wasn't able to take care of them 'cause I was usin'. I was usin' real heavy too." For Marie, contracting HIV was the impetus to get clean and stay off the streets: "I said, 'It's time for me to stop, I'm not indestructible like I thought I was.' So I did stop. I have relapsed, maybe every four or five months it has happened, but I don't put myself in that situation like I did before." The stress of mothering three children without assistance or support often spurred relapses: "To me it starts by getting depressed and then the problems with my kids' father and then the kids. It's like I don't know, I just end up doing it." However, Marie explained that if she can abstain from drugs she will be okay because when she is clean she is able to spend more time with her children. Marie reported that she has been more involved with her children since her diagnosis and is currently concentrating on regaining custody of them.

Illness, especially one that has not yet compromised functional ability, is easier to incorporate into their biographies than separation from their children. Women explained that dealing with the feelings of failure and guilt that result from losing their children transcends the challenges associated with HIV/AIDS. In Nancy's words, "You get to a point [where] you get carried away for so many years that you don't really care about yourself, you don't really care what happens to you, but [to] everybody else."

Drug Use and HIV: The Intersection of Substance Use and Other Conditions

As noted, the majority of women in this study sample have drug-use histories (n = 25, 68 percent) and eighteen of these women (72 percent) used intravenous drugs. As will be demonstrated, substance abuse was responsible for, or at least related to, many of their predicaments, including HIV/AIDS.

Pat contracted HIV when she was eighteen years old. At age twenty-seven she lives alone, has never married, and has no children. Prior to finding out she had HIV infection, Pat was "runnin' the street." Reflecting on her life on the streets, Pat expressed that those times were more disruptive than having HIV has been:

> I think being out in the streets is worse [and more] dangerous. Plus, I didn't have a place to live, can't clean up like I'm used to, you don't eat. I was gettin' seven hundred dollars [a month] and it was gone in one day just gettin' high, drinkin' . . .

Similarly, prior to contracting HIV, Karen described a number of assaults on her identity which culminated in her drug addiction. Among the earliest assaults was her forced separation from her family at the age of thirteen. In an attempt to help their "troubled" daughter, Karen's parents institutionalized her. She described this horrifying experience:

> When I was [thirteen years old] I was put in and out of the diagnostic center . . . and then I was sent to a place for a year. . . . It's a therapeutic community. I was supposed to be there till I was eighteen just because I was a runaway, and the judge told my mother that I was out of control. But when I got there, it was like being in a boot camp. . . . They put you over chairs with thick paddles that have holes in them to make welts on you. . . . It was horrible, horrible; there was brainwashing. As a matter of fact,

years ago they found out the place was corrupt and they closed it down.

She continued to describe that phase of their life:

> I was living on the streets, staying in motel rooms after I dated people for money—not eating, you know; I lived on the street. I was like a homeless person. . . . And I worked for a madam. . . . It was a crazy life. I don't believe it today [when] I look at myself.

When thinking about HIV relative to all she has endured, Karen said, "It doesn't bother me as much as my childhood bothered me. And [HIV/AIDS], that's death, so my childhood was traumatic for me."

Five respondents (14 percent) pointed out the interconnectedness of disruptive events in their lives. These women were well aware of the synergistic effects of previous events, and pondered the question about the relative disruption of HIV more deeply. Even in the midst of her "risky" lifestyle Michelle could not believe that she was addicted to heroin, living in cars, stealing from those she loved, and selling her body for drug money:

> I didn't even know myself—it came to the point where I didn't even know myself. I would look in the mirror and be like, why? I couldn't believe I was doin' the things that I was doin' because it just wasn't me. I mean, I never thought when I was goin' to high school and livin' with my very first boyfriend that two years later I was gonna be stickin' needles in my arm and goin' to prison. And livin' on the streets and out of my cars and not takin' showers for days. I just couldn't imagine that I was doing that when I had so many dreams and so much potential.

Within two years Michelle became addicted to heroin and contracted HIV. At age twenty-eight, Michelle had the virus for seven years at the time of this study and has been clean for a couple of months. She described the interconnection of events:

> Oh, God, it's like all in one, you know what I mean? Like all that goes together. You know that whole two years, it's like one whole nightmare, everything just was like overlapping, the whole, everything.

Rachel, who in the early phases of her illness was afraid to hold her daughter for fear of infecting her, has had her share of assaults on her identity, including cocaine addiction and involvement in violent relationships. In fact, she moved to the Northeast with her daughter to get away from the violent man who gave her HIV. Rachel very clearly explained how the physical abuse, drug addiction, and HIV infection are interconnected through the string of "poor choices" she had made:

> All those difficult times led up to that, to me making that dumb choice. I mean, it's not like one choice—"Oh, I won't have him use a condom tonight." No, it's just a gradual thing because that's why you always have to be on the alert. It's easy for me to say this now, but you always have to. You can't say, well, last Thursday I didn't use a condom, but I used it ever since then. No, you can't do that, 'cause that Thursday could have done it. So, it's like you make mistakes over and over and over and you're bound to get slapped in the face with reality, and I guess that's what happened.

Rachel clearly takes responsibility for her actions, as she sees her behavior as having put her at risk for contracting HIV. Few women, in fact, directly expressed that they were responsible for contracting HIV via their histories of substance abuse. Jessica is one such woman:

> Well, at this point . . . it's been ten years I dealt with it, I came to reality. I'm a realist-type person. . . . I did this to myself. This is the consequence of my actions ten years ago, or whatever how many years ago. That's just life, you know? It's like if I smoke and found out I had cancer. Well, I smoked, so that's the realism to it. . . . I've had crises in my life, but I really can't pinpoint which one was worse than the other. I can go back to finding out when I was HIV positive and how I felt then; it felt bad. But then I can go back to when I was a kid and my mother and father got divorced. It felt bad, you know what I mean?

Several women in this sample wanted others to recognize that being HIV positive is only one part of their personhood. Rachel felt very strongly about, and was most articulate in expressing, her desire for others to see past the HIV infection and see *her*—as a woman, as a mother, as a friend, as someone with other needs and concerns. As

Rachel narratively reconstructed her self-representation, she emphasized her desire to move beyond a stigmatized identity:

> Everything I feel now is not because of HIV; like I'd like to talk to somebody about my problems and not tell them about HIV! Because I have problems anyway. I've had them before; I still do. It's like, "Oh, she's HIV positive. That's why. . . ." I wanted to get some counseling a couple of years ago and I went to this health center. . . . I told them I did a little drugs [and] I feel depressed. And then I had mentioned that I was HIV positive as an afterthought. Well, once I said that, I guess the red light went ding, ding, ding—"Oh, we'll refer you to this HIV specialist." I was like, "Never mind." I didn't want to talk about that; that really didn't bother me, even though they said, "Oh, it stems from that." I had problems before. People have problems that aren't infected. Don't treat me like that; I don't want to be labeled, please. There's other things. I worry about being a good mother. I'm worried about a lot of things! Geez. I'm normal, I have to do things! Shit! Because I don't want to put that in every other part of my life. No!

Other respondents also highlighted the synergistic effects of their behavior. For example, an alcoholic, Robyn knows well the struggles of cleaning up her act. Compared to her battle with alcoholism, HIV did not cause a profound rupture in her life. Prior to becoming infected, Robyn had become accustomed to sickness, uncertainty, and disorder:

> You know, our hearts are extremely tough, because the kind of torture that we put ourselves through with the wear and tear on the body that the alcohol causes, not to mention recuperating and just making ourselves get up and go to work when anyone else would call in sick . . . and then, of course, in the back of my mind even though I never consciously thought much about it, if I did I'd drown it with some alcohol. . . . There was nobody to turn to, you know? Those years were very hectic, just chaos, just total chaos all the time.

In addition to HIV and alcoholism, Robyn has cancer. It is unclear whether the cancer is HIV related, but her need for surgery made the threat of cancer more real and immediate than that of HIV. In particular the physical violation of surgery posed a more serious barrier to her forming a coherent life story:

> I've had this ongoing cancerous thing that they're treating me for and the surgery they were gonna do was a vulvectomy. I don't know if you know what that means. . . . You know what the vulva are? Well, chop 'em off. So to some extent they did that. It's not quite as mutilating as it sounds, but that was the thing that got me, more than the HIV diagnosis was that facing this—this surgery that I felt was mutilating.

Later in the interview, Robyn speculated on HIV relative to cancer and surmises that the cancer was more alarming than HIV:

> [The cancer is] more traumatic. Although, I don't know if it is because I kinda just may have been sorta [in] a little bit of denial even about the HIV. But then there was the period of about six months where I was like really just having a wake for myself; that was it, my life was over, blah, blah, blah, blah. . . . And that only lasted about six months 'cause I'm naturally optimistic and a positive sort of person so that didn't last too long. And then I finally got a grip so I just slapped myself silly and got to work.

As she continued speaking about her cancer, she thoughtfully wove a new strand into her self-analysis. She asserted that HIV infection and cancer are symptoms of her primary problem, alcoholism:

> The worst time in my life is the—the worst thing I ever had—the worst illness I have is the alcoholism. Even to this day, HIV or not, cancer or not, the worst disease I have is alcoholism . . . because it affects your behavior, and it affects your judgment. And when your judgment is impaired you don't make good decisions, you don't take care of yourself. And you feel like a piece of doo-doo, so it takes away your ability to care for yourself.

She continued:

> The HIV was an opportunistic infection of my alcoholism. See, when you think about HIV and the opportunistic infections that come with that because your immune system has weakened. But when your emotional system is weakened, your spiritual self is

weakened, then you do things [and] you don't use good judgment. You don't take care of yourself and then the HIV was able to take hold. So it is an opportunistic infection of the alcoholism, and so for that reason, the alcoholism and my behavior during those years is what . . . was bad. That was the shame, but not the HIV itself; that was just an opportunistic infection.

Substance abuse was tied to some of the worst experiences in these women's lives—they hurt loved ones, stole money, were often ostracized by their families, worked the streets as prostitutes, lost custody of their children, and contracted HIV. As they reflected on these times in their lives, they were quick to note how socially isolated they were and, indeed, socially inept. In retrospect, many felt "less than"—a phrase used by a few of the women in this study to describe their lowered self-esteem. Jessica summarized the view of many former drug addicts:

> Like a year ago sitting here talking to me compared to now is much different. Well, my head, my way of dealing with everyday people all the time is much more right now than it was, say, six months or a year ago. I wasn't in with the real world. I was scared of the real world. You were—I shied away from you because of the fact I felt I was *less than,* you know? Now I feel as equal, so I'm right there with everybody else's level but when you're getting high you're always at a different level. You look different, you act different, you're a totally different person.

Other Traumatic Events

Four women (11 percent) cited other traumatic life events that, in hindsight, they deemed more disruptive than HIV infection, such as the death of loved ones, fighting bureaucracy, and life changes such as divorce. For example, in retrospect, Gina reports that securing supplemental security income (SSI) benefits and applying for U.S. citizenship have caused her great grief, and she tends to think about her illness as a similar hurdle:

> I guess it is a day-by-day thing, you know? You get the day where you get a problem and that's the worst that can happen to you. Then after a while you look back and say, "Well, that wasn't that bad after all." And I guess HIV is the same, but you learn to live with it and, you know, it becomes part of your life.

Failed marriages were also extremely disruptive for a few respondents. For instance, Carol does not have a drug-use history, nor was she ever involved in a violent intimate relationship. She was, however, unhappy with her marriage and longed for something more. Having married at age sixteen, being a wife and mother was all Carol knew. When she courageously decided to get a divorce after being married for ten years, Carol was unprepared for being head of household. She was a displaced homemaker who had no marketable skills, and the thought of immersing herself in the world outside of the home was incredibly frightening:

> Divorce, with two small children, that was a living hell. Actually, emotionally I fell apart a lot worse with that than I did this . . . I was a stay-at-home mother so I really had no skills so that was a *tremendous* change in my life. . . . I was terrified. I had done *nothing*. And two small kids to come home to with all the stress and added responsibility and then the bickering with him. He was constantly angry with me because [in his view] I ruined the family life. . . . [Divorce] was harder on me. I mean, I had to get on nerve pills for a short while. I mean, I wasn't thinking straight. I'd put my wallet in the refrigerator, shit like that. Like, oh, my God, I'm losing my mind! So I didn't get that bad with [HIV infection].

Rose similarly reported that her divorce was perhaps more disruptive than HIV as she, too, was unprepared for living on her own:

> I think the HIV was bad, but when I think about it, probably when my marriage broke up, 'cause I was young, I was like sixteen when I was married. We were married for sixteen years and I was madly in love, and that's all I knew, so I was devastated. And then I was, you know, I went through a really bad time. I had the breakdown. I was cryin' all the time and calling him up. . . . I would say that was like the worst of my life.

* * *

HIV has replaced cancer as the most dreaded disease of our time (Sontag 1989). The terms *HIV* and *AIDS* typically conjure images of loss, mental and physical deterioration, and untimely death. At diagnosis, respondents equated HIV/AIDS with despair and death, and several wanted to take their own lives. Yet, in hindsight, these women do not evaluate HIV infection as the most disruptive event in their lives thus far. For many women who have had to contend with extended periods of violence, drug addictions, other hardships, and illness, even a virulent one, HIV/AIDS diagnosis is reconstructed into a less severe event.

"NOTHING COMPARES TO HIV"

Unlike respondents who viewed HIV as less disruptive than other crises, some women ($n = 10$, 27 percent) concentrated on the losses associated with HIV/AIDS and the possible or probable future complications. These women were touched by other serious assaults (e.g., violence and drug use), but, in retrospect, these events were not insurmountable. In fact, many had overcome these hardships and have been leading "normal" lives. Although violence and drug use certainly can be fatal, the bottom line for these women was that they were not. On the other hand, they viewed AIDS as a guaranteed death sentence. These women highlighted the difficulties of living with HIV/AIDS in Chapter 3. At the risk of repetition, these issues are revisited as it is clear that some respondents interpreted them as difficulties associated with HIV/AIDS while others viewed them as factors underlying the profound rupture caused by the virus, making HIV infection the most disruptive event in their lives thus far.

Death and Dying

Most women for whom HIV is the most disruptive event cited deterioration and mortality as the primary reasons for their assessment. Many feared "the pain and suffering, and everything else that goes with it." Some women were not afraid of death, but dying is another matter. As noted, Hillary, who was diagnosed in 1995, is particularly concerned with how becoming sick will affect her body. Knowing well that AIDS is often accompanied by severe physical manifestations (e.g., wasting and skin problems), she worries that her former healthy-looking self will be lost.

In addition to the physical effects of the virus, women worried about unfulfilled dreams and goals. For women who have never married and do not have any children, for example, the threat of premature death may cause a particularly severe rupture to their identities. As discussed in the first chapter, for women such as Stephanie who could not conceive of becoming pregnant now that she has HIV infection the disruption is particularly profound. Stephanie explained the tension between her desire to have children and her beliefs regarding childbearing among HIV-positive women:

> Well, I thought about it, but I can't really do it. I mean, I could have a child, but I just don't think it would really be right for the child. I mean, sometimes I have really crazy ideas. I mean, the idea of having a child kinda overtakes you occasionally, you know? It's like sometimes you're unaware—you see a really cute baby or a kid and it's sort of like a really physical feeling that you suddenly have that desire. For me, it's really physical, and at that moment it's the only thing you want.

Stephanie became very emotional as she talked about the obstacles HIV/AIDS poses to becoming a mother:

> Then, if you have a baby, are you gonna be there for it? I could probably have a baby, sure, but if I live for another five years then somebody else has to do that. I just don't think it would really be fair. . . . I know in a sense even with all [I've been through] that I would be a lot better than some parents. . . . I think that I could be a good parent, but I don't know if you're a good parent if you have a baby that might possibly be born with a serious illness or you die shortly after it's born.

For some respondents, death and dying are relatively recent preoccupations. Before Alicia contracted HIV infection, she was a single parent struggling to provide a decent home for her son. Fortunately, Alicia lived with her parents who were very supportive and allowed her to work without having to place her son in day care—an option that was neither financially nor normatively feasible. Because Alicia did not experience the assaults that many of the other women did, she considers HIV to be the most disruptive event she has ever faced. This view of the virus, however, is relatively recent. In fact, although she was diagnosed about seven years prior to this study, she pondered the seriousness of her condition only recently:

I've had a good life, ever since, you know, childhood till now. And then besides, you know, I mean the [HIV] bothered me when the medicine started kicking in . . . believe it or not, it didn't click until maybe like a year ago, when I had to start taking meds. You know what I mean? I knew I had it. [But it didn't affect me] 'cause I didn't have to do nothing. I was still living a normal life, until I had to take medicine twice a day. And then that kicked in. And then last month I went to the doctors, my viral load was down and my T-cell count was up, but she wants to keep it that way, she wants to get my viral load undetectable so that means she had to put [me] on protease inhibitors, and then it really kicked in. I was like, "Oh, shit!" When I found out that I had to take the meds, then I said, "Alicia, you gotta start taking care of yourself." I mean, I'm doing it. I got coupons and I went to the health food store.

Similarly, Laurie considered HIV and the prospect of death as the most disruptive factor in her life. Unlike Stephanie and Alicia, however, Laurie also endured violence and poverty. Describing what her life was like before she contracted HIV, Laurie said:

What eventually ended up happening was that they ended up raiding the downstairs apartment for drugs. I had never saw a raid in my life and that scared me, so I went into a shelter. . . . My life was all right. It was hectic, but it was, you know, worthwhile. You know what I mean? I had a purpose; I had things to do, places to go, people to see. And when I went into the shelter my self-esteem was like really, really low. Then I met up with somebody who eventually gave me the virus. But I mean my— my whole life growing up was—my mother was an alcoholic and, of course, she'd wake me up at 2:00 in the morning with the beatings.

Laurie had some trouble articulating her thoughts but was able to convey the relative meaning of HIV infection in her life. In the end, she noted that the other assaults to her sense of self pale in comparison to death and dying: "Nothing compares to it. Nothing compares to knowing that I could die, you know? . . . Everything else is like, I can deal with it."

Loss of Intimacy

Jennifer was diagnosed with HIV ten years prior to this study and now has AIDS. At forty-five years old, she has never married and has no children. Jennifer is college educated, and she has spent most of her career as a high school teacher. Prior to contracting HIV, Jennifer was working two jobs and had a happy and active familial and social life. She described herself as a happy-go-lucky woman. Holding two jobs and maintaining an active social life took its toll, however, and in an attempt to help her meet these responsibilities Jennifer turned to cocaine. In her view, her drug use did not cause any major problems and she was basically satisfied with her life. The only thing missing was a significant other with whom to share it. Because establishing an intimate relationship was so important for Jennifer, HIV was very disruptive. In discussing why HIV was the most disruptive event in her life thus far, Jennifer noted the barriers HIV posed to establishing intimate relationships, especially the difficulty of disclosing her HIV-positive status:

> Well, frankly, I don't feel like I'm desirable by all men now, so it has affected me in that area, and this is why I shelter myself. . . . Like I won't walk into a bar, a restaurant, or a gathering or anything and see a nice-looking man that I'm attracted to, I will not zero in. And normally I would because I'm a very outgoing person . . . [but] he might like me, and then I'm gonna have to get down to tell him, and I don't want to do that.

Not surprisingly, women who have experienced rejection were particularly reticent to become sexually involved. Thalia was initially not afraid to disclose her HIV status, but upon doing so she experienced rejection and does not want to go through it again. She is thirty-two years old, divorced, and has two young sons. A vivacious woman, Thalia is still very interested in forming an exclusive sexual relationship, but HIV may make this impossible. She was dating a man for a few months before she told him she was infected. When she told him, "He seemed fine with it." She has not heard from him since, however. She said, "It didn't go over so well, he has a problem with it. . . . [Relationships] are confusing, the breaks are always there. I don't want to go through it again."

THE RELATIVE IMPACT OF ASSAULTS

The literature regarding women and HIV/AIDS notes that this population—poor, minority, and/or drug addicted (active or recovering)—has had to contend with many assaults on self (e.g., Battle 1997; Bradley-Springer 1994; Flanigan 1995; Jenkins and Coons 1996; O'Donnell 1996). Thus, HIV infection may be just another event in an ongoing string of disruptive events. Indeed, the results of this study support this view to some extent. Not all the women, however, experienced, interpreted, and evaluated their situation in the same way. Several factors appear to be central to women's differential assessment of HIV in relation to other disruptive events including race, drug-use and abuse histories, social support (i.e., presence of, and responses from, individuals in their informal networks), length of time living with HIV, and diagnosis (see Table 7.1). Given the relatively small and nonrandom nature of this sample, these numbers are intended to help illustrate the factors contributing to women's differential assessments, rather than to support broader generalizations.

Racial background appears to contribute to women's differential evaluations, particularly in regard to being a woman of color. Of the African-American and Latina women in my sample, 71 percent said that other assaults were more disruptive than HIV/AIDS compared to 29 percent who reported HIV was more disruptive. White women were split more equally among the two categories (44 percent and 57 percent, respectively). As noted earlier, these results may reflect the effects of marginalization in the lives of women of color. Although many of the white women in this sample have experienced poverty, rejection, and discrimination primarily related to their social class status and lifestyles, they have racial privilege.

Life as a drug addict is a breeding ground for other assaults, such as violence, poverty, homelessness, poor familial relations, or abandonment (e.g., Weissman and Brown 1996; Zierler 1997). Women in this sample described recovering from a drug addiction as being on a roller coaster—getting clean, relapsing, and starting the detox process all over again. Women with substance-abuse histories were more likely than women without substance-abuse histories to say that other assaults on self were more disruptive than HIV infection (68 percent and 32 percent, respectively). The effect of drug use is more marked among those with intravenous drug-use histories; that

TABLE 7.1. Relative Impact of HIV/AIDS

	HIV as most disruptive (%)	Other assaults more disruptive (%)
Race		
White women	43 (*n* = 10)	57 (*n* = 13)
Women of color	29 (*n* = 4)	71 (*n* = 10)
Substance use		
Yes	32 (*n* = 8)	68 (*n* = 17)
No	50 (*n* = 6)	50 (*n* = 6)
IVDU history		
Yes	28 (*n* = 5)	72 (*n* = 13)
No	47 (*n* = 9)	53 (*n* = 10)
History of abuse		
Yes	31 (*n* = 5)	69 (*n* = 11)
No	43 (*n* = 9)	57 (*n* = 12)
Disclosure reaction		
Positive	31 (*n* = 10)	69 (*n* = 22)
Negative	75 (*n* = 3)	25 (*n* = 1)
Know other PWAs		
Yes	31 (*n* = 9)	69 (*n* = 20)
No	71 (*n* = 5)	29 (*n* = 2)
Spouse/significant other		
Yes	20 (*n* = 3)	80 (*n* = 12)
No	50 (*n* = 11)	50 (*n* = 11)
Years HIV positive		
1-5 years	46 (*n* = 5)	54 (*n* = 6)
6-15 years*	35 (*n* = 9)	65 (*n* = 17)
Diagnosis		
HIV positive	34 (*n* = 11)	66 (*n* = 21)
AIDS	60 (*n* = 3)	40 (*n* = 2)

*The "6-10 years" and "11-15 years" categories were combined into one category as there was only one respondent who has been living with HIV for more than ten years.

is, 72 percent of women who used injection drugs said other assaults were more disruptive than HIV infection, and 28 percent believed HIV was more disruptive.

As previously demonstrated, involvement in abusive relationships was often seen as more disruptive than HIV. Assessing their health as basically good (i.e., the absence of debilitating symptoms or opportunistic infections), violence was a greater threat to the women's physical and psychological well-being. In fact, of those who have histories of abuse, 69 percent said that other assaults were more disruptive than HIV infection (versus 31 percent who said HIV was more disruptive).

As discussed in Chapter 5, the relationship between social support and psychological well-being is well established. Thus, we would expect positive social support to have a mediating effect on the disruption caused by HIV. Reactions from others, knowing other individuals with HIV/AIDS, and the presence of a spouse/significant other, are all indicators of the support garnered by women with HIV. Few women ($n = 4$) reported receiving a negative reaction or being abandoned by family and friends upon disclosing their HIV status. Of those who received more positive reactions, though, nearly 70 percent reported that other assaults on self were more disruptive than HIV. Thus, it is likely that the support from significant others helped these women to cope with HIV/AIDS. Of the few women who received mostly negative reactions from others, three quarters reported HIV as having the most profound effects on their lives.

Knowing other individuals who are also infected with HIV also appears to influence women's assessments. That is, respondents who have family members or friends who are HIV positive are more likely to view other assaults as more disruptive than HIV. Knowing others with the virus may help women cope with their illness by alleviating feelings of difference and, hence, restore feelings of normalcy. Although it was not articulated by most of the women in this sample, they may also provide information regarding disease etiology and treatment.

Given the health benefits of having a confidant or other source of positive support (Gupta and Korte 1994), it is not surprising that the presence of a spouse or significant other colors women's perceptions of the disruptive nature of HIV/AIDS. The vast majority of the women involved in a monogamous, intimate relationship at the time of the interview reported that other assaults were more disruptive than HIV infection.

The length of time women had been living with HIV also appears to be related to these differences, especially for those who had been infected for over five years at the time of the study. That is, of those who had been living with HIV infection for six to fifteen years, 65 percent reported that other assaults were more disruptive than HIV (35 percent indicated HIV is more disruptive). Women who had HIV infection for one to five years, however, were more evenly split among the two categories (i.e., 46 percent said HIV has been the most disruptive and 54 percent said it was not). The longer women had been living with HIV, the more likely they were to have integrated it into their biography. Given that many women expected to become sick and/or die soon after they received their diagnosis, the women who have gone a longer time without contracting full-blown AIDS may reassess HIV as less of a threat to their health. Women who were diagnosed more recently, especially within a couple of years of the study, may still expect their health to deteriorate quickly.

Developing full-blown AIDS also appears to influence women's perceptions of the disruptive nature of their illness. Clearly, not being classified as having AIDS may be psychologically comforting. That is, given that AIDS signifies a hastening of deterioration and more severe health problems, these women may experience less anxiety surrounding their illness and may be more hopeful that they may maintain their asymptomatic or relatively well status. The small number of respondents with an AIDS diagnosis ($n = 5$) makes it more difficult to evaluate diagnosis as a key factor in women's appraisals. However, these findings suggest that women who have AIDS may be more likely than their HIV-positive counterparts to view their illness as most problematic.

The ways in which women evaluate the disruption caused by HIV and the factors that influence women's assessments have important implications. First, these results underscore the importance of treating women with cultural sensitivity (e.g., Giachello 1996; Land 1994; Reid 2000; Williams 1995). Given that there appear to be racial differences in the ways women experience and interpret HIV/AIDS, health care professionals need to be cognizant of these differences in approaching the care and treatment of women. Support group facilitators who work with women of color, for example, must be aware of these differences to deal effectively with women's issues, which are apt to go beyond HIV/AIDS. In addition, this knowledge may help minimize conflict in groups that could arise from women's differing backgrounds and experiences.

Second, these results illustrate the importance of social support in coping with illness. More specifically, these findings highlight the significance of relational resources in coping with HIV infection (Bury 1982). In the course of their illness trajectories, the support provided by informal others helped lesson the blow of HIV/AIDS in most instances. As discussed in Chapter 5, however, the unwillingness and/ or inability of potential caregivers to provide emotional and instrumental support in later stages of the disease may cause women to rely more heavily on formal services rather than informal networks.

Last, these findings suggest that women may underestimate the effects and progression of HIV infection, which may lead to non-compliance with treatment protocols and other health-promoting activities (e.g., proper nutrition, rest, and exercise). Moreover, their assessments may lead to less concern with practicing safe sex, which further compromises their health and the health of others.

This analysis underscores the influence of social context on women's assessments of illness. Negative life events, such as substance abuse and violence as well as disadvantaged status, may abate the impact of HIV/AIDS. Women who have had more positive situations in the past, on the other hand, assess HIV infection as more problematic. These factors also may influence their illness behavior, either positively or negatively. For example, Catalan et al. (1996) found that, among women with HIV infection, poor social adjustment and experiencing multiple adverse events were associated with higher psychological morbidity. This result points to the importance of psychosocial care for women with HIV/AIDS and suggests paying close attention to women's experiences outside of HIV. Professionals treating women with HIV/AIDS cannot adequately address the health and social needs of this population without paying attention to women's diverse social milieus and needs. Although there are indeed commonalities across women's experiences, treating them as a homogeneous group will interfere with optimal care and service provision.

Chapter 8

Disruption and Repair: Lessons from Women's Illness Experiences

Over the past two decades AIDS has engendered tremendous social and public health problems. Globally, millions of women are infected with HIV. In the United States, women constitute the fastest-growing AIDS population. To help fill the gap in the social science literature regarding HIV-positive women's illness experience, this research has explored how women experience biographical disruption and mend fractured selves. Thus, the previous chapters have shown the ways in which women interpret and manage their illness as a disruptive event. This chapter will elaborate on the effects their illness has had on their identities, discuss the nature and consequences of women's coping styles, address the broader issues related to living with HIV/AIDS, and discuss the theoretical and practical implications of this research.

THE STRENGTHS AND WEAKNESSES OF WOMEN'S COPING

Employing biographical disruption as an analytic framework to interpret and present women's experiences with HIV/AIDS highlights the meanings they attach to HIV/AIDS, the psychosocial effects of illness, and the resources they tap to cope and accomplish legitimation (Bury 1982). As demonstrated in Chapter 2, when women first learned that they were HIV positive most felt hopeless and uncertain of how they would manage with their illness. In addition to deterioration and death, women worried that their illness would negatively affect their social worlds. Thus, issues regarding intimate relationships and economic survival, for instance, were highlighted as important concerns. Internalizing the negative stereotypes surrounding HIV/ AIDS, women felt unworthy of positive attention from others. Further, women who had worked to turn their lives around by abstaining from drugs and getting job training, for example, felt as if the virus had robbed them of their second chance to pursue socially legitimate endeavors. Despite women's initial reactions, however, most have incorporated HIV infection into their lives, thereby minimizing disruption. As the women's narratives reveal, a disease that initially symbolized a premature end to their hopes and dreams has been largely reconstructed into a crisis with positive consequences.

As with the respondents in Barroso's (1997a) study, the women in this study first viewed HIV/AIDS as a threat, then as a challenge, and ultimately as an identity-building experience. The knowledge that their time is limited caused many women to rethink their lives and to try to make changes that, before their diagnosis, appeared less urgent (e.g., abstaining from drugs and strengthening social ties). Much of this change has entailed a reformulation of how they approach everyday living. To make the most out of a tragic situation, women worked to gain greater control over their lives. They accomplished this by relying on supportive relational resources, including their families, support groups, and projects designed to further AIDS awareness and education. Many women were introduced to these groups and projects through their health care providers. In addition to informal others, therefore, formal networks also helped them incorporate their illness into their lives and maintain their identity, or accomplish legitimation. Through their interaction with others, they felt more socially connected and began to view themselves, and hence HIV, in more positive terms. Women's reconstruction is more clearly demonstrated in Chapter 7, as many women revealed that their social environments had exposed them to other assaults on self (i.e., violence, poverty, mother/child separation, substance abuse, and marital dissolution), which are more disruptive than HIV/AIDS.

Despite women's apparent "success," some respondents' reconstructed assessments of HIV/AIDS are problematic. Although the women have reconstructed HIV into a less disruptive event and have thereby minimized losses of self, their actions reveal ways in which they have not adjusted well. Perceiving HIV as less dangerous than they originally thought, women may give priority to other issues and pay less attention to their health. For example, women who have not developed debilitating symptoms may be less likely to adopt healthier habits, or, conversely, abstain from harmful behaviors, such as drug use. Continued intravenous drug use has been shown to accelerate disease progression and to interfere with adherence to treatment regimens (Campbell 1990; Selwyn, O'Connor, and Schottenfeld 1995). Moreover, continued needle sharing increases the risk of transmission. Protected sex is also critical to help protect others from contracting HIV as well as ensuring that women are not exposed to a different, more lethal, strain of the disease. As noted, fewer than half of this sample (41 percent) reported practicing safe sex regularly. Thus, although women expressed having a greater understanding of HIV/AIDS, many appear to underestimate the seriousness of the virus.

Further, women's narratives reveal contradictions between their positive adjustment and unrealistic rationales for their progress. For example, although many reported greater self-esteem because they are living relatively well with their illness, their belief that they can overcome their illness (e.g., fight illness progression or "get better") also demonstrates some degree of denial. With new strains of the virus proving resistant to relatively recent antiretroviral therapies, it may become more difficult for women to believe they can win their fight against HIV/AIDS. Women's reluctance to legally appoint a guardian(s) for their children may also reflect denial. Interestingly, women who reported coming to terms with their mortality had not prepared for the welfare of their children. As mothers, it is harder for these women to deal with their children's hardships than with their own health. Knowing that illness or death may stop them from fulfilling their protective, nurturing roles is very unsettling. Perhaps contributing to their anxiety is the fact that most of these women, upon their deaths, do not have spouses or significant others who will assume responsibility for their children. The inability to fulfill roles such as mothering is an undeniable blow to a woman's sense of self, and thus they may avoid guardianship issues to maintain their identities as mothers.

These contradictions may be due, in part, to respondents attempting to represent their "best selves" to the interviewer. Thus, it is possible that these women tried to portray a more positive view of themselves despite HIV. Inconsistency of self, although potentially problematic, is largely unavoidable. As Ewing (1990) notes, individuals may experience a continuous identity despite shifts in self. Thus, these women may seek, and attempt to present, coherent selves, but their conceptions are altered by their present situations. Women's "interpretive reconstructions" (Grove 1992) of their experiences, then, are bound to demonstrate inconsistencies, especially among women who have faced dramatically altered situations.

Factors Affecting Women's Coping Strategies

Women's ways of coping demonstrate positive and negative approaches to HIV/AIDS. Strategies that entail active efforts at mediating stressors are more effective than those that are not problem focused. Going public and being involved in activist efforts helped some women obtain social support and gain knowledge about their illness and available services. Ideally, support groups, which serve a similar function, also allow women to share their experiences in a confidential, nonjudgmental environment.

Given the effectiveness of different coping strategies, it is important to note the factors that may impact women's choices of repair strategies. Intravenous drug use affects women's reactions to their diagnoses and may negatively affect the nature of their helping networks. Similarly, these women have presumably less experience in adopting healthy coping styles. As noted in Chapter 4, compared to women who have not used intravenous drugs, women with histories of intravenous drug use in this sample were more likely to engage in avoidance and denial, and were less likely to report making positive health and lifestyle changes. Women who did not use intravenous drugs, on the other hand, were more likely than nonusers to be engaged in activist efforts and to identify spirituality as a coping resource.

Length of time since diagnosis also appears to influence women's coping styles. Relative to women who received their diagnosis within six years prior to this study, women who have been living with HIV infection for seven or more years (an interval by which many individuals develop symptoms and/or progress to AIDS) were more likely to have gone public with their illness. These women were also more likely to report making positive lifestyle changes and strengthening religious or spiritual ties. Women who have been living with HIV for fewer than seven years, on the other hand, were more likely to engage in avoidance/denial than women who received their diagnosis more than seven years prior.

The presence of a partner may also impact women's coping strategies. Of women who were involved in AIDS activism, for example, nearly 60 percent did not have a significant other. The vast majority of women who credited support groups with helping them cope were not involved in a romantic relationship (86 percent). Women who did not have a partner were also more likely than those involved in an intimate relationship to strengthen or renew spiritual ties as a way of coping. The presence of a significant other may also hinder women from making positive lifestyle changes. The fact that many of these women's partners engage in substance abuse and are therefore less likely to engage in healthy habits themselves might help explain this finding.

Women's Informal Networks and Coping with HIV/AIDS

Health and illness are couched in social relations; thus, the response of individuals in the women's social networks was critical to their interpretation of HIV/AIDS. Issues regarding fear of stigma, rejection, and abandonment loomed large for these women (see Chapter 3). Women who were not involved in a romantic relationship at the time of the interview were more likely to highlight fear of rejection, problems establishing intimate relations, and death and dying. The presence of a significant other, then, may help assure women that they are accepted and may help alleviate the fear associated with premature death. Similarly, women living with HIV infection for seven or more years were also more likely to highlight these issues compared to women who have been HIV positive for less than seven years. These women may have had more time to experience the consequences of HIV and, thus, are less optimistic regarding the impact of HIV on their daily lives.

Although these fears have subsided, in part, due to familial and peer acceptance, the stability of women's networks is questionable. In terms of feeling better about themselves, women credited their familial networks with helping them incorporate HIV/AIDS into their biographies. In particular, the emotional support provided by women's parents, children, and significant others have facilitated their repair work. Here again, women may have overstated the positive role of their networks in order to present an ideal self-representation. As noted in Chapter 5, instrumentally, women's informal networks have been less dependable, and women continue to support and care for others despite their compromised health status. In addition, intravenous drug use and length of time since diagnosis may also affect the nature of women's informal support networks. The majority who reported having supportive familial networks did not have intravenous drug-use histories. Women who did not have intravenous drug-use histories were also more likely to emphasize the positive contributions their children made to their repair process. In fact, three-quarters of the women who described instances of negative support (e.g., lack of assistance, love, or emotional support) have intravenous drug-use histories. Thus, women who have used intravenous drugs may have greater difficulty mobilizing positive informal support networks and, hence, be more vulnerable to unmet need for informal support.

In terms of years living with HIV infection, three-quarters of women who described instances of negative support have been living with HIV for seven or more years, suggesting that positive support may corrode over the course of one's illness. Family members who were initially supportive may be unwilling or unable to provide emotional support continuously. This is an especially troubling finding given that the vast majority of these women are asymptomatic and have not called on their networks for more intense caregiving tasks.

Women's relationships with those in their informal networks further illustrates how women's multiple roles and responsibilities increase their levels of "vicarious stress" (i.e., stress stemming from crises in the lives of loved ones) (Thomas 1997). Respondents' concerns regarding the health, well-being, and financial situation of their children and/or lovers contributed to distress. Although assuming responsibility for the welfare of others was a major way in which women retained participation in meaningful, identity-reaffirming social roles, it also has negative consequences, such as having less time and energy to devote to their own well-being.

Clearly, caregiving for other ill individuals is a pertinent example of the vicarious stress many HIV-positive women experience. In Chapter 6, it is shown how caring both positively contributes to women's sense of self and poses difficulties for women striving to tend to their own health. As HIV/AIDS continues to increase among heterosexual populations, women are more likely to assume the role of primary caregiver (Wight, LeBlanc, and Aneshensel 1998). In addition, as gay HIV-infected men's partners become too ill to be primary caregivers, mothers and sisters will become their primary caregivers in greater numbers (Wight, LeBlanc, and Aneshensel 1998).

FORMAL CARE AND WOMEN
WITH HIV INFECTION

Given the tenuous nature of women's networks, women may be more apt to turn to formal sources for care when the need arises. These women may have to contend with fragmented and uncoordinated medical and social services, impeding the quality and continuity of care for themselves as well as their ability to care for others (ACT UP 1990; Rodriguez-Trias and Marte 1995; Russell and Smith 1998; Stein et al. 2000). Chronically ill mothers in other studies have complained that health care services often do not accommodate their dual needs as people with chronic health problems and as mothers (Thorne 1990). Similarly, lacking a holistic approach to care, formal services for women with HIV/AIDS are often inadequate, particularly for women with children (Kaspar 1989; Schuster et al. 2000; Weitz 1993). Service programs, for instance, are often insufficient for HIV-positive mothers because few agencies offer support groups for children or housing/residential programs specifically for people with HIV/AIDS. In order to obtain safe and adequate housing, mothers must often give up custody of their children (Weitz 1993). Ignoring the value attached to women's roles as mothers and the ways in which children help women cope, services for people with HIV/AIDS cannot sufficiently address women's needs.

Although the problems with health and social services for HIV-positive women have been highlighted in other research (e.g., Rodriguez-Trias and Marte 1995; Russell and Smith 1998; Weitz 1993), the vast majority of respondents in this study were very satisfied with their medical care. They were particularly pleased by the attention they received from their care providers, especially their physicians. Overall, respondents believed they were getting the best medical care available. When asked about the services they received, women enthusiastically described their medical encounters. They revered their providers because they treated them with respect, listened to their concerns, and validated their experiences. As Donna explained:

> They're very great, that's why I'll recommend [them] for anyone. I mean, they don't think about your color, they don't care about what you got, they [are] just there to help you . . . they were even gonna come to the house and talk to my son for me . . . they're so wonderful. I could never have [been in] a better hospital. I know I'm in good hands. . . . All the doctors treat you with much, much respect; that's what I like about the doctors.

A couple of women did express having trouble obtaining dental care; however, most could not think of ways to improve the services they received because they have had such positive experiences and little difficulty accessing services. A couple of women discussed organizational changes that would benefit most women with HIV/AIDS. These women have negotiated the system with few problems in large part because they were fairly knowledgeable and/or had assistance getting referred to services. Thus, they spoke about creating a system that was accessible to women who are not well linked and may lack the knowledge to access the services they need. For example, Robyn explained that she is in a unique position because she is employed, has health insurance, and is aware of the resources available to her. She worries, however, about women who lack the resources and assistance required to get their needs met:

> I know that there are a lot of people that don't have these things. And a lot of people fall through the cracks because they don't have money or they can't reach out. Or maybe they're still very active in their addictions, and so unless that illness is treated and got under control you can't treat the other thing; it's just useless. That's what bothers me, is that there's a lot of people that have a lot of needs that aren't being filled.

Related to Robyn's point, Gina remarked:

> I think there should be more a client-oriented [approach] . . . like the social services. It should more pay attention to what the client wants and needs. I think they should pass out a questionnaire and ask what you want. Not, you know, make decisions and do

the things [because] there's too much bureaucracy and there are snobbish people.

Gina cited the Massachusetts-based AIDS coalition as a fine example of how organizations that serve HIV-positive women can help them gain a voice as care consumers:

> You go there, you get trained to be an advocate to speak with the media, to do all those things you have to go to speak with the legislator. They teach you how to write a letter properly, so you can be listened to.

Other women pointed out that services need to make a greater effort to disseminate information about HIV/AIDS to the general public. As Geraldine said:

> They seem adequate, I just don't know that everybody knows enough about it. Like I know I'm all set, but I don't know that the man on the street knows, the general person. There's a lot of ignorance out there. You know, the services may be great, but there's still a lot of people with attitude and ignorance that really need some serious educating.

EMPOWERMENT AND SOCIAL CHANGE

AIDS crystallizes women's inequality and powerlessness. Empowering women to gain control of their lives is critical to the quality of women's lives. Programs and outreach efforts directed toward empowering women are imperative for prevention efforts as well. Moreover, relatively simple and inexpensive vehicles such as support groups may help to reach out to women. More important, support groups cultivate social consciousness and foster AIDS activism (Lather and Smithies 1997). Of course, empowerment is obstructed by women's social and economic status; thus, broader societal changes are also needed. If the women who are infected with HIV/AIDS were not predominately members of marginalized groups, the social and epidemiological consequences would be different. Poor access to adequate health services and poorer health prior to infection, for example, would be eased by greater social and economic resources. As Travers and Bennett (1996:70) note, HIV/AIDS exacerbates the marginalization of women:

> The lack of political, economic, legal, societal, and personal power that typifies the position of women in so many cultures has resulted in negative consequences for women living with HIV/AIDS. Consequences of disempowerment include isolation, stigma, discrimination and neglect, because the powerless are rendered ineffective and voiceless.

Thomas (1997:552) points out that "facilitating empowerment begins with assisting clients to develop a critical awareness of their situation and enabling them to master their environment to achieve self-determination." Nearly three-quarters of the sample analyzed in this text have taken part in empowering projects at some point in their lives. They have, for example, become involved in education and prevention efforts that have advanced their knowledge of HIV/AIDS and elucidated their status as women with HIV/AIDS. Women's involvement in support groups has also facilitated a critical awareness of the plight of women with HIV infection. Participation in activist-oriented organizations has validated their experiences and, in turn, promoted positive senses of self. These assets, greater understanding and self-esteem, are fundamental resources in empowerment. Indeed, to a certain extent some women have formed collective identities around their illness (Carricaburu and Pierret 1995). For example, several respondents discussed their experiences in a collective voice; that is, they talked about "women with AIDS," about "minority women," and about "women with substance-abuse problems." However, women with AIDS have not cultivated the same degree of collective consciousness as their gay male counterparts. As discussed in Chapter 4, many factors impede women's collective participation, including race and class differences. In addition, women's involvement may be curtailed by structural barriers such as a lack of knowledge regarding how to join support groups and the difficulty of securing child care and transportation. However, the findings of this research suggest that these vehicles may be more effective at validating women's experiences than disseminating greater knowledge of the epidemiological aspects of HIV infection and prevention.

EXPERIENCING ILLNESS: EXTENDING HIV-POSITIVE WOMEN'S EXPERIENCES TO OTHER POPULATIONS

Employing a narrative approach, this study provides insight into the multifaceted nature of HIV-positive women's lives. Using a convenience sample, however, it is not possible to present data that reflect the lived experiences of the most vulnerable women living with HIV/AIDS. The nonrandom nature of this sample also raises questions about the representativeness of results for other populations. As is evident, the nature of this sample may be unique in that these women were fairly well linked to medical services, and a fairly large proportion of them were actively involved in AIDS-related causes. This may, in part, account for the articulate nature of the women in this sample. That is, having experience discussing their situations with others, they have become skilled in communicating their stories and concerns. Indeed, they may even have internalized ideal types of HIV narratives. Study replication is essential to determine whether the results of this analysis are applicable to people with HIV/AIDS in other settings. This sample also does not adequately represent the experiences of women of color. Research that concentrates on minority women is also needed in order to better serve the largest, and most vulnerable, female AIDS population. Last, although many women in this sample reported having some symptoms, such as fatigue and gynecologic infections, most did not report debilitating conditions. Women who have debilitating symptoms or who are functionally impaired are faced with further obstacles in everyday living and identity maintenance. When faced with serious health problems, the issues HIV-positive women identified in Chapter 3 will likely be revised. Thus, research that investigates how women interpret and cope with HIV at various points in their illness trajectories is needed. Longitudinal research would demonstrate how women's perceptions of their illness, support networks, and coping strategies change over time. Further research that investigates the influence of key variables (e.g., intravenous drug use, years since diagnosis, and presence of a spouse/partner) on women's coping efforts is also needed.

Women with HIV infection are a unique illness population—they have a disease that is sexually transmitted and fatal, they are over-represented by marginalized populations, and many have (or are associated with others who have) histories of illicit behavior. These factors invoke far less social tolerance and sympathy than that given to other illness populations. As a group, they may also be less likely to have a positive support network.

In applying Bury's (1982) disruption and repair framework to women's experiences with HIV, we have an opportunity to see how theory fits when people have had histories of crisis. Relative to other illness populations, the theory may be less applicable to people who have prior illness experiences or other hardships that have altered their biographies (Pound, Gompertz, and Ebrahim 1998). In particular, this is likely to be the case for poor, marginalized women who are not well linked to health and social services. Nevertheless, we can adapt elements of biographical disruption and repair to help investigate how women with HIV/AIDS examine their life circumstances.

Despite the unique situation of women with HIV, research into their experiences with HIV may provide insight into the study of how other populations experience and manage illness. By examining how women respond to, and cope with, HIV/AIDS, this research contributes to illness literature exploring the ways in which individuals respond and cope when they receive a diagnosis of a terminal illness (Barroso 1997a). Other researchers, such as Charmaz (1983b), have emphasized the losses associated with chronic illness, including diminished senses of self and strained relationships (Lindsey 1996). In this study, it has also been demonstrated how HIV infection has caused identity problems and negatively affected relationships. Knowledge of the negative effects of managing a chronic illness is important because it helps us to understand the psychosocial sequelae of illness. However, by also concentrating on the positive elements of illness adaptation, we get a more complete picture of the complex impact illness has on people's lives. As discussed in this text, these beneficial aspects of illness do not necessarily translate into positive coping strategies, but they do influence women's sense of self. Although this may seem contradictory, indeed people's lives and their adaptations to illness are often so. If we search only for unified and coherent selves we will rarely find them. Just as people's lives are not linear, neither are their adaptations to illness.

These findings underscore the importance of people's lived experiences of health and illness and the social contexts in which they occur. These findings also underscore the complexity surrounding the impact of negative life events on the individual's sense of self (Thoits 1995b). Analyses of the individual's subjective experiences, or insider's perspectives, provide a more comprehensive understanding of women's experiences with HIV/AIDS. It is especially important to give a voice to the most marginalized illness populations as these individuals are often silenced and their health and social needs go unmet. Indeed, they have a great deal to teach us about living with illness.

Appendix

Sample Demographic Summary

Name	Age	Race	Marital Status	Education	Employment	Children < 18	Years Living with HIV Infection
Adele	47	white	divorced	<HS	no	0	6
Alicia	34	black	never married	HS/GED	yes	2	7
Becky	47	white	separated	some college	yes	0	7
Carmen	29	Latina	never married	<HS	no	3	6
Carolyn	47	white	divorced	HS/GED	yes	0	4
Dawn	37	white	never married	HS/GED	no	0	10
Debra	41	black	never married	some college	no	1	13
Denise	38	black	never married	HS/GED	no	1	7
Donna	43	black	never married	HS/GED	yes	0	3
Geraldine	40	white	divorced	HS/GED	yes	0	9
Gina	33	white	divorced	some college	no	0	6
Heather	38	white	married	HS/GED	yes	0	10
Hillary	54	white	widowed	HS/GED	yes	0	8
Irene	60	Latina	divorced	College	no	0	6
Jennifer	45	white	divorced	College	no	0	10
Jessica	31	white	divorced	<HS	yes	2	10

Jocelyn	44	black	never married	<HS	no	1	2
Julia	45	white	widowed	some college	yes	0	7
Karen	32	white	divorced	<HS	no	1	10
Kelly	48	white	divorced	Associates/ trade school	no	0	5
Kim	34	black	divorced	<HS	no	2	9
Kristen	39	black	never married	Associates/ trade school	no	0	3
Laurie	39	white	divorced	HS/GED	yes	2	6
Lisa	35	white	separated	Associates/ trade school	no	1	9
Marie	31	black	never married	Associates/ trade school	no	2	6
Melissa	27	white	divorced	HS/GED	no	2	3
Michelle	28	white	never married	some college	no	0	7
Nancy	40	white	divorced	Associates/ trade school	no	0	5
Pat	32	white	never married	<HS	no	3	4
Rachel	32	Latina	never married	Associates/ trade school	no	1	7
Robyn	48	white	divorced	Associates/ trade school	yes	0	7
Rose	49	white	divorced	some college	yes	0	6
Sheila	38	black	married	some college	yes	2	8
Shirley	47	black	never married	HS/GED	no	0	6
Stephanie	38	white	never married	some college	no	0	8
Thalia	32	white	divorced	some college	yes	2	3
Valerie	40	black	married	Associates/ trade school	no	0	2

References

Abel, E. 1990. *Who Care for the Elderly? Public Policy and the Experiences of Adult Daughters.* Philadelphia: Temple University Press.

ACT UP. 1990. *Women, AIDS and Activism.* Boston: South End Press.

Adelman, M. 1989. Social Support and AIDS. *AIDS and Public Policy Journal* 4:31-39.

Alford-Cooper, F. 1993. Women as Family Caregivers: An American Social Problem. *Journal of Women and Aging* 5:43-57.

Allen, S.M. 1994. Gender Differences in Spousal Caregiving and Unmet Need for Care. *Journal of Gerontology* 49:S187-S195.

Allen, S.M., Goldscheider, F., and Ciambrone, D. 1999. Gender roles, Marital intimacy, and Nomination of Spouse as Primary Caregiver. *The Gerontologist* 39: 150-158

Altschuler, J. 1993. Gender and Illness: Implications for Family Therapy. *Journal of Family Therapy* 15:381-401.

Andersen, M.L. 1993. *Thinking About Women: Sociological Perspectives on Sex and Gender.* New York: Macmillan.

Anderson, D., Deshaies, G., and Jobin, J. 1996. Social Support, Social Networks and Coronary Artery Disease Rehabilitation: A Review. *Canadian Journal of Cardiology* 12:739-744.

Andrews, S., Williams, A.B., and Neil, K. 1993. The Mother-Child Relationship in the HIV-1 Positive Family. *IMAGE: Journal of Nursing Scholarship* 25:93-198.

Antonucci, T.C. and Akiyama, H. 1987. An Examination of Sex Differences in Social Support Among Older Men and Women. *Sex Roles* 17:737-749.

Arber, S. and Ginn, J. 1991. *Gender and Later Life.* London: Sage.

Avants, K.S., Warburton, L.A., and Margolin, A. 2001. Spiritual and Religious Support in Recovery from Addiction among HIV-Positive Injection Drug Users. *Journal of Psychoactive Drugs* 33:39-45.

Baker, S., Sudit, M., and Litwak, E. 1998. Caregiver Characteristics and the Types of Assistance Provided by Caregivers to Minority Women Living with HIV/AIDS. *Journal of Cultural Diversity* 5:11-18.

Barroso, J. 1997a. Reconstructing My Life: Becoming a Long-Term Survivor of AIDS. *Qualitative Health Research* 7:57-74.

Barroso, J. 1997b. Social Support and Long-Term Survivors of AIDS. *Western Journal of Nursing Research* 19:554-582.

Barusch, A.S. and Spaid, W.M. 1989. Gender Difference in Caregiving: Why Do Wives Report Greater Burden? *The Gerontologist* 30:667-676.

188 *WOMEN'S EXPERIENCES WITH HIV/AIDS*

Batt, S. 1992. Breast Cancer Epidemic: Two Women's Personal Views. *Propaganda Review* 9:14-16.

Battle, S. 1997. The Bond Is Called Blackness: Black Women and AIDS. In N. Goldstein and J.L. Manlowe (Eds.), *The Gender Politics of HIV/AIDS in Women* (pp. 282-301). New York: New York University Press.

Becker, G. 1997. *Disrupted Lives: How People Create Meaning in a Chaotic World*. Los Angeles: University of California Press.

Becvar, D.S. 1996. I am a Woman First: A Message About Breast Cancer. *Families, Systems and Health* 14:83-88.

Beder, J. 1995. Perceived Social Support and Adjustment to Mastectomy in Socioeconomically Disadvantaged Black Women. *Social Work in Health Care* 22:55-71.

Belgrave, F.Z. and Lewis, D.M. 1994. The Role of Social Support in Compliance and Other Health Behaviors for African Americans with Chronic Illnesses. *Journal of Health and Social Policy* 5:55-68.

Belkin, G.S., Fleishman, J.A., Stein, M.D., Piette, J., and Mor, V. 1992. Physical Symptoms and Depressive Symptoms Among Individuals with HIV Infection. *Psychosomatics* 33:416-427.

Berkman, L.F. and Syme, L.S. 1979. Social Networks, Host Resistance, and Mortality: A Nine-Year Follow-Up Study of Alameda County Residents. *American Journal of Epidemiology* 109:186-204.

Bigby, C. 1997. Parental Substitutes? The Role of Siblings in the Lives of Older People with Intellectual Disability. *Journal of Gerontological Social Work* 29:3-21.

Bix, A.S. 1997. Diseases Chasing Money and Power: Breast Cancer and AIDS Activism Challenging Authority. *Journal of Policy History* 9:5-32.

Bonuck, K.A. 1993. AIDS and Families: Cultural, Psychosocial, and Functional Impacts. *Social Work in Health Care* 18:75-89.

Bradley-Springer, L.A. 1994. Reproductive Decision-Making in the Age of AIDS. *IMAGE: Journal of Nursing Scholarship* 26:241-246.

Brander, P. and Norton, V. 1993. *Women Living with HIV/AIDS: Issues and Needs Confronting Women with HIV/AIDS and Women Who Care for People with HIV/AIDS*. Manatu Hauora: Ministry of Health.

Brody, E.M. 1981. "Women in the Middle" and Family Help to Older People. *The Gerontologist* 21:471-479.

Brook, D.W., Brook, J.S., Whiteman, M., Roberto, J., Masci, J.R., Amundsen, F., and de Catalogne, J. 1999. Coping among HIV-negative and HIV-positive female injection drug users. *AIDS Education and Prevention* 11:262-273.

Brook, J.S., Brook, D.W., Win, P.T., Whiteman, M., Masci, J.R., de Catalogne, J., Roberto, J., and Amundsen, F. 1997. Coping with AIDS. A Longitudinal Study. *American Journal of the Addictions* 6:11-20.

Brown, P. 1991. Themes in Medical Sociology. *Journal of Health Politics, Policy and Law* 16:595-604.

Brown, S.N. 1996. Clinical and Psychosocial Issues of Women with HIV/AIDS. In A. O'Leary and L.S. Jemmott (Eds.), *Women and AIDS: Coping and Care* (pp. 151-166). New York: Plenum Press.

Bunting, S.M. 2001. Sustaining the Relationship: Women's Caregiving in the Context of HIV Disease. *Health Care for Women International* 22:131-148.

Bury, J. 1995. Women and HIV/AIDS: Medical Issues. In L. Doyal, J. Naidoo, and T. Wilton (Eds.), *AIDS Setting a Feminist Agenda* (pp. 30-41). London: Taylor and Francis.

Bury, M. 1982. Chronic Illness As Biographical Disruption. *Sociology of Health and Illness* 4:167-182.

Bury, M. 1991. The Sociology of Chronic Illness: A Review of Research and Prospects. *Sociology of Health and Illness* 13:451-468.

Campbell, C.A. 1990. Women and AIDS. *Social Science and Medicine* 30:407-415.

Carlson, G.C., O'Campo, P., Faden, R.R., and Eke, A. 1997. Women's Disclosure of HIV Status: Experiences of Mistreatment and Violence in an Urban Setting. *Women and Health* 25:19-31.

Carr, E.W. and Morris, T. 1996. Spirituality and Patients with Advanced Cancer: A Social Work Response. *Journal of Psychosocial Oncology* 14:71-81.

Carricaburu, D. and Pierret, J. 1995. From Biographical Disruption to Biographical Reinforcement: The Case of HIV-Positive Men. *Sociology of Health and Illness* 17:65-88.

Catalan, J., Beevor, A., Cassidy, L., Burgess, A.P., Meadows, J., Pergami, A., Gazzard, B., and Barton, S. 1996. Women and HIV Infection: Investigation of its Psychosocial Consequences. *Journal of Psychosomatic Research* 41:39-47.

Catz, S.L., Kelly, J.A., Bogart, L.M., Benotsch, E.G., and McAuliffe, T.L. 2000. Patterns, Correlates, and Barriers to Medication Adherence Among Persons Prescribed New Treatments for HIV Disease. *Health Psychology* 19:124-133.

Centers for Disease Control and Prevention (CDC). 1998. *HIV/AIDS Surveillance Report* 9:1-37. Atlanta: U.S. Department of Health and Human Services.

Centers for Disease Control and Prevention (CDC). 1999. Fact Sheets, HIV/AIDS Among U.S. Women: Minority and Young Women at Continuing Risk. Accessed online <http://www.cdc.gov>.

Chamberlin, J. 1978. *On Our Own: Patient-Controlled Alternatives to the Mental Health System*. New York: Hawthorn Books.

Charmaz, K. 1983a. The Grounded Theory Method: An Explication and Interpretation. In R.M. Emerson (Ed.), *Contemporary Field Research* (pp. 109-126). Belmont: Wadsworth.

Charmaz, K. 1983b. Loss of Self: A Fundamental Form of Suffering in the Chronically Ill. *Sociology of Health and Illness* 5:168-195.

Charmaz, K. 1987. Struggling for a Self: Identity Levels of the Chronically Ill. In J.A. Roth and P. Conrad (Eds.), *Research in the Sociology of Health Care* (pp. 283-321). Greenwich, CT: JAI Press.

Charmaz, K. 1991. *Good Days, Bad Days: The Self in Chronic Illness and Time.* New Jersey: Rutgers University Press.

Charmaz, K. 1994. Identity Dilemmas of Chronically Ill Men. *Sociological Quarterly* 35:269-288.

Chung, J.Y. and Magraw, M.M. 1992. A Group Approach to Psychosocial Issues Faced by HIV-Positive Women. *Hospital and Community Psychiatry* 43:891-894.

Connidis, I.A. 1994. Sibling Support in Older Age. *Journal of Gerontology* 49: S309-S317.

Conrad, P. 1986. The Social Meaning of AIDS. *Social Policy* 17:51-56.

Conrad, P. 1987. The Experience of Illness: Recent and New Directions. In J.A. Roth and P. Conrad (Eds.), *Research in the Sociology of Health Care* (pp. 1-31). Greenwich, CT: JAI Press.

Corbin, J.M. and Strauss, A. 1987. Accompaniments of Chronic Illness: Changes in Body, Self, Biography, and Biographical Time. In J.A. Roth and P. Conrad (Eds.), *Research in the Sociology of Health Care* (pp. 249-281). Greenwich, CT: JAI Press.

Corbin, J.M. and Strauss, A. 1988. *Unending Work and Care: Managing Chronic Illness at Home.* San Francisco: Jossey-Bass, Inc.

Corea, G. 1992. *The Invisible Epidemic.* New York: HarperCollins.

Coward, D.D. 1994. Meaning and Purpose in the Lives of Persons with AIDS. *Public Health Nursing* 11:331-336.

Crystal, S. and Sambamoorthi, U. 1996. Care Needs and Access to Care Among Women Living with HIV. In L. Sherr, C. Hankins, and L. Bennett (Eds.), *AIDS as a Gender Issue: Psychosocial Perspectives* (pp. 191-196). London: Taylor and Francis.

Crystal, S. and Schiller, N.G. 1993. Stigma and Homecoming: Family Caregiving and the "Disaffiliated" Intravenous Drug User. In G.L. Albrecht and R. Zimmerman (Eds.), *Advances in Medical Sociology: The Social and Behavioral Aspects of AIDS* (pp. 165-184). Greenwich, CT: JAI Press.

Dane, B.O. 1991. Anticipatory Mourning of Middle-Aged Parents of Adult Children with AIDS. *Families in Society* 72:108-115.

DeGenova, M.K., Patton, D.M., Jurich, J.A., and MacDermid, S.M. 1994. Ways of Coping Among HIV-Infected Individuals. *Journal of Social Psychology* 134:655-663.

Demi, A., Moneyham, L., Sowell, R., and Leland, C. 1997. Coping Strategies Used by HIV-Infected Women. *Omega: Journal of Death and Dying* 35:377-391.

DeRidder, D., Karlein, T.D., and Schreurs, M.G. 1996. Coping, Social Support and Chronic Disease: A Research Agenda. *Psychology, Health and Medicine* 1:71-82.

do-Rozario, L. 1997. Spirituality in the Lives of People with Disability and Chronic Illness: A Creative Paradigm of Wholeness and Reconstitution. *Disability and Rehabilitation* 19:427-434.

Douglas, P.H. and Pinsky, L. 1996. *The Essential AIDS Fact Book.* New York: Pocket Books.

Dowling, S. 1995. Women Have Feelings Too: Mental Health Needs of Women Living with HIV Infection. In L. Doyal, J. Naidoo, and T. Wilton (Eds.), *AIDS Setting a Feminist Agenda* (pp. 113-121). London: Taylor and Francis.

Dunbar, H.T., Mueller, C.W., Medina, C., and Wolf, T. 1998. Psychological and Spiritual Growth in Women Living with HIV. *Social Work* 43:144-154.

El-Bassel, N. and Schilling, R.F. 1994. Social Support and Sexual Risk Taking Among Women on Methadone. *AIDS* 6:506-513.

Ell, K., Nishimoto, R., Mediansky, L., Mantell, J., and Hamovitch, M. 1992. Social Relations, Social Support and Survival Among Patients with Cancer. *Journal of Psychosomatic Research* 36:531-541.

Epstein, S. 1995. The Construction of Lay Expertise: AIDS Activism and the Forging of Credibility in the Reform of Clinical Trials. *Science, Technology, and Human Values* 20:408-437.

Ewing, K.P. 1990. The Illusion of Wholeness: Culture, Self, and the Experience of Inconsistency. *Ethos* 18:251-278.

Flanigan, T. 1995. AIDS in the Circle of Life. *Signs and Symptoms* 19:13-14.

Florence, M.E., Lutzen, K., and Alexius, B. 1994. Adaptation of Heterosexually Infected HIV-Positive Women: A Swedish Pilot Study. *Health Care for Women International* 15:265-273.

Foley, M., Skurnick, J.H., Kennedy, C.A., Valentin, R., and Louria, D.B. 1994. Family Support for Heterosexual Partners in HIV-Serodiscordant Couples. *AIDS* 8:1483-1487.

Folkman, S., Chesney, M.A., and Christopher-Richards, A. 1994. Stress and Coping in Caregiving Partners of Men with AIDS. *Psychiatric Clinics of North America* 17:35-53.

Ford, M.E., Tilley, B.C., and McDonald, P.E. 1998. Social Support Among African-American Adults with Diabetes. *Journal of the National Medical Association* 90:425-432.

Forstein, M. and McDaniel, J.S. 2001. Medical Overview of HIV Infection and AIDS. *Psychiatric Annals* 31:16-20.

Friedland, J., Renwick, R., and McColl, M. 1996. Coping and Social Support As Determinants of Quality of Life in HIV/AIDS. *AIDS Care* 8:15-31.

Friedman, S.R., Des Jarlais, D.C., and Sterk, C.E. 1990. AIDS and the Social Relations of Intravenous Drug Users. *Milbank Quarterly* 68:85-110.

Friedman, S.R., Richard Curtis, M.S., Neaigus, A., and Des Jarlais, D.C. 1992. Organizing Drug Users Against AIDS. In J. Huber and B.E. Schneider (Eds.), *The Social Context of AIDS* (pp. 115-130). Newbury Park: Sage.

Fuller, R.L., Geis, S.B., and Rush, J. 1988. Lovers of AIDS Victims: A Minority Group Experience. *Death Studies* 12:1-7.

Fullilove, M.T., Fullilove, R.E., Haynes, K., and Gross, S. 1990. Black Women and AIDS Prevention: A View Towards Understanding the Gender Rules. *The Journal of Sex Research* 27:47-64.

Giachello, A.L. 1996. Latino Women. In M. Bayne-Smith (Ed.), *Race, Gender and Health* (pp. 121-171). Thousand Oaks, CA: Sage.

Gielen, A.C., McDonnell, K.A., Wu, A.W., O'Campo, P., and Faden, R. 2001. Quality of Life Among Women Living with HIV: The Importance of Violence, Social Support, and Self Care Behaviors. *Social Science and Medicine* 52:315-322.

Gielen, A.C., O'Campo, P., Faden, R.R., and Eke, A. 1997. Women's Disclosure of HIV Status: Experiences of Mistreatment and Violence in an Urban Setting. *Women & Health* 25:19-31.

Gilligan, C. 1982. *In a Different Voice.* Cambridge, MA: Harvard University Press.

Gillman, R.R. and Newman, B.S. 1996. Psychosocial Concerns and Strengths of Women with HIV Infection: An Empirical Study. *Families in Society* 77:131-141.

Goffman, E. 1963. *Stigma.* Englewood Cliffs, NJ: Prentice-Hall.

Goggin, K., Catley, D., Brisco, S.T., Engelson, E.S., Rabkin, J.G., and Kotler, D.P. 2001. A Female Perspective on Living with HIV Disease. *Health and Social Work* 26:80-89.

Gordillo, V., del-Amo, J., Soriano, V., and Gonzalez-Lahoz, J. 1999. Sociodemographic and Psychological Variables Influencing Adherence to Antiretroviral Therapy. *AIDS* 13:1763-1769.

Graham, H. 1983. Caring: A Labour of Love. In J. Finch and D. Groves (Eds.), *A Labour of Love: Women, Work, and Caring* (pp. 13-30). London: Routledge and Kegan Paul.

Grassi, L., Caloro, G., Zamorani, M., and Ramelli, E. 1997. Psychological Morbidity and Psychosocial Variables Associated with Life-Threatening Illness: A Comparative Study of Patients with HIV Infection or Cancer. *Psychology, Health and Medicine* 2:29-39.

Green, G. 1993. Editorial Review: Social Support and HIV. *AIDS Care* 5:87-104.

Green, G. 1996. Stigma and Social Relationships of People with HIV: Does Gender Make a Difference? In L. Sherr, C. Hankins, and L. Bennett (Eds.), *AIDS As a Gender Issue: Psychosocial Perspectives* (pp. 46-63). London: Taylor and Francis.

Greenberg, J.B., Johnson, W.D., and Fichtner, R.R. 1996. A Community Support Group for HIV-Seropositive Drug Users: Is Attendance Associated with Reductions in Risk Behavior? *AIDS Care* 8:529-540.

Grove, K. 1992. Change and Identity: Nurse Practitioners' Accounts of Occupational Choice. *Current Research on Occupations and Professions* 7:141-155.

Grummon, K., Rigby, E.D., Orr, D., Procidano, M., and Reznikoff, M. 1994. Psychosocial Variables that Affect the Psychological Adjustment of IVDU Patients with AIDS. *Journal of Clinical Psychology* 50:488-502.

Gupta, G.R. and Weiss, E. 1993. Women's Lives and Sex: Implications for AIDS Prevention. *Culture, Medicine and Psychiatry* 17:399-412.

Gupta, V. and Korte, C. 1994. The Effects of a Confidant and a Peer Group on the Well-Being of Single Elders. *International Journal of Aging and Human Development* 39:293-302.

Hackl, K.L., Somlai, A.M., Kelly, J.A., and Kalichman, S.C. 1997. Women Living with HIV/AIDS: The Dual Challenge of Being a Patient and Caregiver. *Health Social Work* 22:53-62.

Hall, B.A. 1997. Spirituality in Terminal Illness. An Alternative View of Theory. *Journal of Holistic Nursing* 15:82-96.

Hart, S., Gore-Felton, C., Maldonado, J., Lagana, L., Blake-Mortimer, J., Israelski, D., Koopman, C., and Spiegel, D. 2000. The Relationship Between Pain and Coping Styles Among HIV-Positive Men and Women. *Psychology and Health* 15:869-879.

Havermans, T. and Eiser, C. 1994. Siblings of a Child with Cancer. *Child Care, Health and Development* 20:309-322.

Heath, J. and Rodway, M.R. 1999. Psychosocial Needs of Women Infected with HIV. *Social Work in Health Care* 29:43-57.

Heckman, T.G., Somlai, A.M., Sikkema, K. J., Kelly, J.A., and Franzoi, S.L. 1997. Psychosocial Predictors of Life Satisfaction Among Persons Living with HIV Infection and AIDS. *Journal of Association of Nurses in AIDS Care* 8:21-30.

Henderson, S. 1992. Living with the Virus: Perspectives from HIV-Positive Women in London. In N. Dorn, S. Henderson, and N. South (Eds.), *AIDS: Women, Drugs and Social Care* (pp. 8-29). London: Falmer.

Herek, G.M. 1999. AIDS and Stigma. *American Behavioral Scientist* 42:1106-1116.

Holland, J., Ramazanoglu, J., Scott, S., Sharpe, S., and Thomson, R. 1990. Sex, Gender and Power: Young Women's Sexuality in the Shadow of AIDS. *Sociology of Health and Illness* 12:336-350.

House, J.S., Landis, K.R., and Umberson, D. 1988. Social Relationships and Health. *Science* 241:540-545.

Jaccard, J.E., Wilson, T.E., and Radecki, C.M. 1995. Psychological Issues in the Treatment of HIV-Infected Women. In H.L. Minkoff, J.A. DeHovitz, and A. Duerr (Eds.), *HIV Infection in Women* (pp. 87-105). New York: Raven Press.

Jenkins, R.A. 1995. Religion and HIV: Implications for Research and Intervention. *Journal of Social Issues* 51:131-144.

Jenkins, S.R. and Coons, H.L. 1996. Psychosocial Stress and Adaptation Processes for Women Coping with HIV/AIDS. In A. O'Leary and L.S. Jemmott (Eds.), *Women and AIDS: Coping and Care* (pp. 33-86). New York: Plenum Press.

Jewett, J.F. and Hecht, F.M. 1993. Preventive Health Care for Adults with HIV Infection. *JAMA* 269:1144-1153.

Johnson, C.L. 1983. Dyadic Family Relations and Social Support. *The Gerontologist* 23:377-383.

Johnston, D., Stall, R., and Smith, K. 1995. Reliance by Gay Men and Intravenous Drug Users on Friends and Family for AIDS-Related Care. *AIDS Care* 7:307-319.

Kadushin, G. 1996. Gay Men with AIDS and Their Families of Origin: An Analysis of Social Support. *Health and Social Work* 21:141-149.

Kaiser Foundation. 2001. Fact Sheet, *Women and AIDS*. Accessed online <http://www.kff.org>.

Kalichman, S.C. and Catz, S.L. 2000. Stressors in HIV Infection. In K.H. Nott and K. Vedhara (Eds.), *Psychosocial and Biomedical Interactions in HIV Infection* (pp. 31-60). Amsterdam, Netherlands: Harwood Academic Publishers.

Kalichman, S.C., Sikkema, K.J., and Somlai, A. 1996. People Living with HIV Infection Who Attend and Do Not Attend Support Groups: A Pilot Study of Needs, Characteristics, and Experiences. *AIDS Care* 8:589-599.

Kaplan, M.S., Marks, G., and Mertens, S.B. 1997. Distress and Coping Among Women with HIV Infection: Preliminary Findings from a Multiethnic Sample. *American Journal of Orthopsychiatry* 67:80-91.

Karon, S. 1991. The Difference It Makes: Caregiver Gender and Access to Community-Based Long-Term Care Services in the Social/HMO. Brandeis, unpublished doctoral dissertation.

Kaspar, B. 1989. Women and AIDS: A Psycho-Social Perspective. *Affilia* 4:7-22.

Katz, M.H., Douglas, J.M., Bolan, G.A., Marx, R., Sweat, M., Park, M.S., and Buchbinder, S.P. 1996. Depression and Use of Mental Health Services Among HIV-Infected Men. *AIDS Care* 8:433-442.

Keller, M. 1998. Psychosocial Care of Breast Cancer Patients. *Anticancer Research* 18:2257-2259.

Kelly, J., Murphy, D.A., Bahr, G.R., and Kalichman, S.C. 1993. Outcome of Cognitive-Behavioral and Support Groups Brief Therapies for Depressed, HIV-Infected Persons. *American Journal of Psychiatry* 150:1679-1686.

Kimberly, J.A. and Serovich, J.M. 1996. Perceived Social Support Among People Living with HIV/AIDS. *American Journal of Family Therapy* 24:41-53.

Klee, H. 1995. Drug Misuse and Suicide: Assessing the Impact of HIV. *AIDS Care* 7:S145-S155.

Kleinman, A. 1988. *The Illness Narratives*. New York: Basic Books.

Koopman, C., et al. 2000. Relationships of Perceived Stress to Coping, Attachment and Social Support Among HIV-Positive Persons. *AIDS Care* 12:663-672.

Krohn, B. 1998. When Death Is Near: Helping Families Cope. *Geriatric Nursing* 19:276-278.

Kutner, N.G. 1987. Social Ties, Social Support, and Perceived Health Status Among Chronically Disabled People. *Social Science and Medicine* 25:29-34.

Lamping, D.L. and Mercey, D. 1996. Health-Related Quality of Life in Women with HIV Infection. In L. Sherr, C. Hankins, and L. Bennett (Eds.), *AIDS As a Gender Issue: Psychosocial Perspectives* (pp. 78-98). London: Taylor and Francis.

Land, H. 1994. AIDS and Women of Color. *Families in Society* 75:355-361.

Lather, P. and Smithies, C. 1997. *Troubling the Angels: Women Living with HIV/AIDS*. Boulder, CO: Westview Press.

Lawless, S., Kippax, S., and Crawford, J. 1996. Dirty, Disease and Undeserving: The Positioning of HIV-Positive Women. *Social Science and Medicine* 43:1371-1377.

Lea, A. 1994. Women with HIV and Their Burden of Caring. *Health Care for Women International* 15:489-501.

Lee, F.R. 1995. For Women with AIDS, Anguish of Having Babies. *New York Times*. May 9, A1:B6.

Leserman, J., Perkins, D.O., and Evans, D.L. 1992. Coping with the Threat of AIDS: The Role of Social Support. *American Journal of Psychiatry* 149:1514-1520.

Levine, C. 1990. AIDS and Changing Concepts of Family. *Milbank Quarterly* 68:33-58.

Levy, A., Laska, F., Abelhauser, A., Delfraissy, J.F., Goujard, C., Boue, F., and Dormont, J. 1999. Disclosure of HIV seropositivity. *Journal of Clinical Psychology* 55:1041-1049.

Lindsey, E. 1996. Health Within Illness: Experiences of Chronically Ill/Disabled People. *Journal of Advanced Nursing* 24:465-472.

Linn, J.G., Lewis, F.M., Cain, V.A., and Kimbrough, G.A. 1993. HIV Illness, Social Support, Sense of Coherence, and Psychosocial Well-Being in a Sample of Help-Seeking Adults. *AIDS Education and Prevention* 5:254-262.

Linn, J.G., Poku, K.A., Cain, V.A., Holzapfel, K.M., and Crawford, D.F. 1995. Psychosocial Outcomes of HIV Illness in Male and Female African-American Clients. *Social Work in Health Care* 21:43-59.

Linsk, N.L. and Poindexter, C.C. 2001. Older Caregivers for Family Members with HIV or AIDS: Reasons for Caring. *Journal of Applied Gerontology* 19:181-202.

Littlewood, B. 1994. Life, Love and HIV: The Women's Symposium on HIV and AIDS. *Critical Social Policy* 14:5-23.

Lugton, J. 1997. The Nature of Social Support As Experienced by Women Treated for Breast Cancer. *Journal of Advanced Nursing* 25:1184-1191.

Lyketsos, C.G., Hoover, D.R., Guccione, M., and Dew, M.A. 1996. Changes in Depressive Symptoms As AIDS Develops. *American Journal of Psychiatry* 153:1430-1437.

Lynch, S.A. 1998. Who Supports Whom? How Age and Gender Affect the Perceived Quality of Support from Family and Friends. *The Gerontologist* 38:231-238.

Magura, S., Siddiqi, Q., Shapiro, J., Grossman, J.I., Lipton, D.S., Marion, I.J., Weisenfeld, L., Amann, K.R., and Koger, J. 1991. Outcomes of an AIDS Prevention Program for Methadone Patients. *The International Journal of the Addictions* 26:629-655.

Mansergh, G., Marks, G., and Simoni, J.M. 1995. Self-Disclosure of HIV Infection Among Men Who Vary in Time Since Seropositive Diagnosis and Symptomatic Status. *AIDS* 9:639-644.

Martin, J.I. and Knox, J. 1997. Self-Esteem Instability and Its Implications for HIV Prevention Among Gay Men. *Health and Social Work* 22:264-273.

Martin, J.L. and Dean, L. 1993. Bereavement Following Death from AIDS: Unique Problems, Reactions, and Special Needs. In M.S. Stroebe, W. Stroebe, and R.O. Hansson (Eds.), *Handbook of Bereavement: Theory, Research and Intervention* (pp. 317-330). Cambridge: University Press.

Maynard, M. and Purvis, J. 1994. *Researching Women's Lives from a Feminist Perspective*. London: Taylor and Francis.

Mellins, C.A., Ehrhardt, A.A., Newman, L., and Conrad, M. 1996. "Selective Kin": Defining the Caregivers and Families of Children with HIV Disease. In A. O'Leary and L.S. Jemmott (Eds.), *Women and AIDS: Coping and Care* (pp. 123-149). New York: Plenum Press.

Melvin, D. 1996. Don't Forget the Children: Families Living with HIV Infection. In L. Sherr, C. Hankins, and L. Bennett (Eds.), *AIDS As a Gender Issue: Psychosocial Perspectives* (pp. 215-234). London: Taylor and Francis.

Meyer, P., Tapley, K., and Bazargan, M. 1996. Depression in HIV Symptomatic Gay and Bisexual Men. *Journal of Gay and Lesbian Social Services* 5:69-85.

Miller, B. and Kaufman, J.E. 1996. Beyond Gender Stereotypes: Spouse Caregivers of Persons with Dementia. *Journal of Aging Studies* 10:189-204.

Millison, M.B. 1995. A Review of the Research on Spiritual Care and Hospice. *Hospice Journal* 10:3-18.

Mishler, E.G. 1992. Work, Identity, and Narrative. In G.C. Rosenwald and R.L. Ochberg (Eds.), *Storied Lives: The Cultural Politics of Self-Understanding* (pp. 21-40). New Haven: Yale University Press.

Moneyham, L., Hennessy, M., Sowell, R., Demi, A., Seals, B., and Mizuno, Y. 1998. The Effectiveness of Coping Strategies Used by HIV-Seropositive Women. *Research in Nursing and Health* 21:351-362.

Moneyham, L., Seals, B., Demi, A., Sowell, R., Cohen, L., and Guillory, J. 1996. Experiences of Disclosure in Women Infected with HIV. *Health Care for Women International* 17:209-221.

Moneyham, L., Sowell, R., Seals, B., and Demi, A. 2000. Depressive Symptoms Among African-American Women with HIV Disease. *Scholarly Inquiry for Nursing Practice* 14:9-39.

Monti-Catania, D. 1997. Women, Violence, and HIV/AIDS. In N. Goldstein and J.L. Manlowe (Eds.), *The Gender Politics of HIV/AIDS: Perspectives on the Pandemic in the United States* (pp. 242-251). New York: New York University Press.

Morokoff, P.J., Mays, V.M., and Coons, H.L. 1997. HIV Infection and AIDS. In S.J. Gallant, G.P. Keita, and E. Royak-Schaler (Eds.), *Health Care for Women: Psychological, Social, and Behavioral Influence* (pp. 273-293). Washington, DC: American Psychological Association.

Moser, K.M., Sowell, R.L., and Phillips, K.D. 2001. Issues of Women Dually Diagnosed with HIV Infection and Substance-Use Problems in the Carolinas. *Issues in Mental Health Nursing* 22:23-49.

Namir, S., Alumbaugh, M.J., Fawzy, I.F., and Wolcott, D.L. 1989. The Relationship of Social Support to Physical and Psychological Aspects of AIDS. *Psychology and Health* 3:77-86.

Nichols, M.L. 1995. Social Support and Coping in Young Adolescents with Cancer. *Pediatric Nursing* 21:235-240.

Nolan, P. and Crawford, P. 1997. Towards a Rhetoric of Spirituality in Mental Health Care. *Journal of Advanced Nursing* 26:289-294.

Nyamathi, A., Flaskerud, J., Leake, B., and Chen, S. 1996. Impoverished Women at Risk for AIDS: Social Support Variables. *Journal of Psychosocial Nursing and Mental Health Services* 34:31-39.

Oakley, A. 1981. Interviewing Women: A Contradiction in Terms. In H. Roberts (Ed.), *Doing Feminist Research* (pp. 136-152). Boston: Routledge and Kegan Paul.

O'Donnell, M. 1996. *HIV/AIDS: Loss, Grief, Challenge, and Hope*. London: Taylor and Francis.

O'Sullivan, S. 1992. Pregnancy, HIV and Women. In S. O'Sullivan and K. Thomson (Eds.), *Positively Women: Living with AIDS* (pp. 235-241). London: Sheba Feminist Press.

Pace, J.C. and Stables, J.L. 1997. Correlates of Spiritual Well-Being in Terminally Ill Persons with AIDS and Terminally Ill Persons with Cancer. *Journal of the Association of Nurses in AIDS Care* 8:31-42.

Pedersen, S.S. and Elklit, A. 1998. Traumatisation, Psychological Defense Style, Coping, Symptomatology, and Social Support in HIV-Positive: A Pilot Study. *Scandinavian Journal of Psychology* 39:55-60.

Penninx, B.W., Van-Tilburg, T., Deeg, D.J., Kriegsman, D.M., Boeke, A.J., and van-Eijk, J.T. 1997. Direct and Buffer Effects of Social Support and Personal Coping Resources in Individuals with Arthritis. *Social Science and Medicine* 44:393-402.

Persson, E. 1994. The Threat of AIDS to the Health of Women. *International Journal of Gynecology and Obstetrics* 46:189-193.

Peterson, J.L., Folkman, S., and Bakeman, R. 1996. Stress, Coping, HIV Status, Psychosocial Resources, and Depressive Mood in African-American Gay, Bisexual, and Heterosexual Men. *American Journal of Community Psychology* 24:461-487.

Pivnick, A. 1994. Loss and Regeneration: Influences on the Reproductive Decisions of HIV-Positive, Drug-Using Women. *Medical Anthropology* 16:39-62.

Pivnick, A., Jacobson, A., Eric, K., Mulvihill, M., Hsu, M.A., and Drucker, E. 1991. Reproductive Decisions Among HIV-Infected, Drug-Using Women: The Importance of Mother-Child Coresidence. *Medical Anthropology Quarterly* 5:153-169.

Pound, P., Gompertz, P., and Ebrahim, S. 1998. Illness in the Context of Older Age: The Case of Stroke. *Sociology of Health and Illness* 20:489-506.

Primomo, J., Yates, B.C., and Woods, N.F. 1990. Social Support for Women During Chronic Illness: The Relationship Among Sources and Types to Adjustment. *Research in Health and Nursing* 13:153-161.

Pruchno, R.A. 1990. The Effects of Help Patterns on the Mental Health of Spouse Caregivers. *Research on Aging* 12:57-71.

Quinn, S.C. 1993. AIDS and the African-American Woman: The Triple Burden of Race, Class, and Gender. *Health Education Quarterly* 20:305-320.

Register, C. 1989. *Living with Chronic Illness: Days of Patience and Passion*. New York: Bantam Books.

Reid, P.T. 2000. Women, Ethnicity, and AIDS: What's Love Got to Do with It? *Sex Roles* 42:709-722.

Reinharz, S. 1992. *Feminist Methods in Social Research*. New York: Oxford University Press.

Richardson, D. 1989. *Women and the AIDS Crisis*. London: Pandora Press.

Rieder, I. and Ruppelt, P. (Eds). 1988. *AIDS: The Women*. San Francisco: Cleis Press.

Riley, J.W. Jr. 1983. Dying and the Meanings of Death: Sociological Inquiries. *Annual Review of Sociology* 9:191-216.

Robinson, I. 1990. Personal Narratives, Social Careers and Medical Courses: Analyzing Life Trajectories in Autobiographies of People with Multiple Sclerosis. *Social Science and Medicine* 30:1173-1186.

Rodgers, A.Y. 1995. The Relationship Between Changes in Sexual Support and Adjustment to AIDS in Gay Males. *Social Work in Health Care* 20:37-47.

Rodriguez-Trias, H. and Marte, C. 1995. Challenges and Possibilities: Women, HIV, and the Health Care System in the 1990s. In B.E Schneider and N.E. Stoller (Eds.), *Women Resisting AIDS: Feminist Strategies of Empowerment* (pp. 299-321). Philadelphia: Temple University Press.

Rosenwald, G.C. and Ochberg, R.L. (Eds.). 1992. *Storied Lives: The Cultural Politics of Self-Understanding*. New Haven: Yale University Press.

Ross, M.W. and Ryan, L. 1995. The Little Deaths: Perceptions of HIV, Sexuality and Quality of Life in Gay Men. *Journal of Psychology and Human Sexuality* 7:1-20.

Rosser, S.V. 1991. Perspectives: AIDS and Women. *AIDS Education and Prevention* 3:230-240.

Russell, J.M. and Smith, K. 1998. HIV-Infected Women and Women's Services. *Health Care for Women International* 19:131-139.

Scharf, E. 1992. Research: HIV/AIDS and the Invisibility of Women. In S. O'Sullivan and K. Thomson (Eds.), *Positively Women: Living with AIDS* (pp. 187-196). London: Sheba Feminist Press.

Schiller, N.G. 1993. The Invisible Women: Caregiving and the Construction of AIDS Health Services. *Culture, Medicine and Psychiatry* 17:487-512.

Schiller, N.G., Crystal, S., and Lewellen, D. 1996. Risky Business: The Cultural Constructions of AIDS Risk Groups. In P. Brown (Ed.), *Perspectives in Medical Sociology*, Second Edition (pp. 707-727). Belmont: Waveland Press, Inc.

Schneider, B.E. 1992. AIDS and Class, Gender, and Race Relations. In J. Huber and B.E. Schneider (Eds.), *The Social Context of AIDS* (pp. 19-43). Newbury Park: Sage.

Schneider, B.E. and Stoller, N.E. (Eds). 1995. *Women Resisting AIDS: Feminist Strategies of Empowerment*. Philadelphia: Temple University Press.

Schneider, J.W. and Conrad, P. 1980. In the Closet with Illness: Epilepsy, Stigma Potential and Information Control. *Social Problems* 28:32-44.

Schreurs, K.M.G. and DeRidder, D.T.D. 1997. Integration of Coping and Social Support Perspectives: Implications for the Study and Adaptation to Chronic Diseases. *Clinical Psychology Review* 17:89-112.

Schuster, M.A., Kanouse, D.E., Morton, S.C., Bozzette, S.A., Miu, A., Scott, G.B., and Shapiro, M.F. 2000. HIV-Infected Parents and their Children in the United States. *American Journal of Public Health* 90:1074-1081.

Selwyn, P.A., O'Connor, P.G., and Schottenfeld, R.S. 1995. Female Drug Users with HIV Infection: Issues for Medical Care and Substance Abuse Treatment. In H.L. Minkoff, J.A. DeHovitz, and A. Duerr (Eds.), *HIV Infection in Women* (pp. 241-291). New York: Raven Press.

Semple, S., Patterson, T.L., Temoshok, L.R., McCutchan, J.A., Straits-Troster, K.A., Chandler, J.L., and Grant, I. 1993. Identification of Pyschobiological Stressors Among HIV-Positive Women. *Women and Health* 20:15-36.

Serovich, J.M., Kimberly, J.A., Mosack, K.E., and Lewis, T. 2001. The Role of Family and Friend Social Support in Reducing Emotional Distress Among HIV-Positive Women. *AIDS Care* 13:335-341.

Shayne, V.T. and Kaplan, B.J. 1991. Double Victims: Poor Women and AIDS. *Women and Health* 16:21-37.

Sherr, L., Petrak, J., Melvin, D., Davey, T., Glover, L., and Hedge, B. 1993. Psychological Trauma Associated with AIDS and HIV Infection in Women. *Counseling Psychology Quarterly* 6:99-108.

Siegel, K., Gluhoski, V.L., and Karus, D. 1997. Coping and Mood in HIV-Positive Women. *Psychological Reports* 81:435-442.

Siegel, K. and Krauss, B.J. 1991. Living with HIV Infection: Adaptive Tasks of Seropositive Gay Men. *Journal of Health and Social Behavior* 32:17-32.

Simoni, J.M. and Cooperman, N.A. 2000. Stressors and Strengths Among Women Living with HIV/AIDS in New York City. *AIDS Care* 12:291-297.

Simoni, J.M., Davis, M.L., Drossman, J.A., and Weinberg, B.A. 2000. Mothers with HIV/AIDS and Their Children: Disclosure and Guardianship Issues. *Women and Health* 31:39-54.

Simoni, J.M. and Ng, M.T. 2000. Trauma, Coping, and Depression Among Women with HIV/AIDS in New York City. *AIDS Care* 12:567-580.

Singh, N., Berman, S.M., Swindells, S., Justis, J.C., Mohr, J.A., Squier, C., and Wagener, M.M. 1999. Adherence of Human Immunodeficiency Virus-Infected Patients to Antiretroviral Therapy. *Clinical Infectious Diseases* 29:824-830.

Smeltzer, S. and Whipple, B. 1991. Women with HIV Infection: The Unrecognized Population. *Health Values* 15:41-48.

Smith, D., Warren, D., Solomon, L., and Schuman, P. 1996. The Design, Participants, and Selected Early Findings of the HIV Epidemiology Research (HER)

Study: A Prospective Cohort Study of the Impact of HIV Infection on the Health of American Women. In A. O'Leary and L.S. Jemmott (Eds.), *Women and AIDS: Coping and Care* (pp. 185-205). New York: Plenum Press.

Smith, E., Redman, R., Burns, T.L., and Sagert, K.M. 1985. Perceptions of Social Support Among Patients with Recently Diagnosed Breast, Endometrial, and Ovarian Cancer: An Exploratory Study. *Journal of Psychosocial Oncology* 3:65-81.

Smith, M.Y. and Rapkin, B.D. 1995. Unmet Needs for Help Among Persons with AIDS. *AIDS Care* 7:353-363.

Somlai, A.M., Kelly, J.A., Wagstaff, D.A., and Whitson, D.P. 1998. Patterns, Predictors, and Situational Contexts of HIV Risk Behaviors Among Homeless Men and Women. *Social Work* 43:7-20.

Songwathana, P. 2001. Women and AIDS Caregiving: Women's Work? *Health Care for Women International* 22: 263-279.

Sontag, S. 1989. *AIDS and Its Metaphors*. New York: Anchor Books.

Sosnowitz, B.G. 1995. AIDS Prevention, Minority Women, and Gender Assertiveness. In J. Huber and B.E. Schneider (Eds.), *The Social Context of AIDS* (pp. 131-161). Newbury Park: Sage.

Sowell, R., Moneyham, L., Hennessy, M., Guillory, J., Demi, A., and Seals, B. 2000. Spiritual Activities As a Resistance Resource for Women with Human Immunodeficiency Virus. *Nursing Research* 49:73-82.

Sowell, R.L., Seals, B.F., Moneyham, L., Demi, A., Cohen, L. and Brake, S. 1997. Quality of Life in HIV-Infected Women in the South Eastern United States. *AIDS Care* 9:501-512.

Stein, M.D., Crystal, S., Cunningham, W.E., Ananthanarayanan, A., Andersen, R.M., Turner, B.J., Zierler, S., Morton, S., Katz, M.H., Bozzette, S.A., Shapiro, M.F., and Schuster, M.A. 2000. Delays in Seeking HIV Care Due to Competing Caregiver Responsibilities. *American Journal of Public Health* 90:1138-1140.

Stein, M.D. and Hanna, L. 1997. Use of Mental Health Services by HIV-Infected Women. *Journal of Women's Health* 6:569-574.

Stevens, P.E. 1996. Struggles with Symptoms: Women's Narratives of Managing HIV Illness. *Journal of Holistic Nursing* 14:142-160.

Stoller, E.P. and Cutler, S.J. 1992. The Impact of Gender on Configurations of Care Among Married Elderly Couples. *Research on Aging* 14:315-330.

Stolley, J.M. and Koenig, H. 1997. Religion/Spirituality and Health Among Elderly African Americans and Hispanics. *Journal of Psychosocial Nursing and Mental Health Services* 35:2-8.

Stone, R., Cafferata, G.L., and Sangl, J. 1987. Caregivers of the Frail Elderly: A National Profile. *The Gerontologist* 27:616-626.

Stowe, A., Ross, M.W., Wodak, A., Thomas, G.V., and Larson, S.A. 1993. Significant Relationships and Social Supports of Injecting Drug Users and Their Implications for HIV/AIDS Services. *AIDS Care* 5:23-33.

Strauss, A.L. and Glaser, B.G. 1975. *Chronic Illness and the Quality of Life*. Saint Louis: Mosby.

Stuntzer-Gibson, D. 1991. Women and HIV Disease: An Emerging Social Crisis. *Social Work* 36:22-27.

Suffet, F. and Lifshitz, M. 1991. Women Addicts and the Threat of AIDS. *Qualitative Health Research* 1:51-79.

Suh,T., Mandel, W., Latkin, C., and Kim, J. 1997. Social Network Characteristics and Injecting HIV-Risk Behaviors Among Street Injection Drug Users. *Drug and Alcohol Dependency* 47:137-143.

Swindells, S., Mohr, J., Justis, J.C., Berman, S., Squier, C., Wagener, M.M., and Singh, N. 1999. Quality of Life in Patients with Human Immunodeficiency Virus Infection: Impact of Social Support, Coping Style and Hopelessness. *International Journal of STD and AIDS* 10:383-391.

Thoits, P.A. 1995a. Identity Relevant Events and Psychological Symptoms: A Cautionary Tale. *Journal of Health and Social Behavior* 36:72-82.

Thoits, P.A. 1995b. Stress, Coping, and Social Support Processes: Where Are We? What Next? *Journal of Health and Social Behavior, Extra Issue* (pp. 53-79).

Thomas, E. 1968. Role Theory, Personality, and the Individual. In E.F. Borgatta and W. Lambert (Eds.), *Handbook of Personality Theory and Research* (pp. 691-727). Chicago: Rand McNally.

Thomas, S.P. 1997. Distressing Aspects of Women's Roles, Vicarious Stresses, and Health Consequences. *Issues in Mental Health Nursing* 18:539-557.

Thompson, S.C. and Pitts, J. 1992. In Sickness and Health: Chronic Illness, Marriage and Spousal Caregiving. In S. Spacapan and S. Oskamp (Eds.), *Helping and Being Helped* (pp. 115-151). Newbury Park, CA: Sage.

Thorne, S.E. 1990. Mothers with Chronic Illness: A Predicament of Social Construction. *Health Care for Women International* 11:209-221.

Travers, M. and Bennett, L. 1996. AIDS, Women and Power. In L. Sherr, C. Hankins, and L. Bennett (Eds.), *AIDS As a Gender Issue: Psychosocial Perspectives* (pp. 64-77). London: Taylor and Francis.

Van-Servellen, G., Sarna, L., and Jablonski, K.J. 1998. Women with HIV: Living with Symptoms. *Western Journal of Nursing Research* 20:448-464.

Ventis, W.L. 1995. The Relationships Between Religion and Mental Health. *Journal of Social Issues* 51:33-48.

Vincke, J. and Bolton, R. 1994. Social Support, Depression, and Self-Acceptance Among Gay Men. *Human Relations* 47:1049-1062.

Wachter, R.M. 1992. AIDS, Activism, and the Politics of Health. *New England Journal of Medicine* 326:128-133.

Ward, M.C. 1993. A Different Disease: HIV/AIDS and Health Care for Women in Poverty. *Culture, Medicine and Psychiatry* 17:413-430.

202   *WOMEN'S EXPERIENCES WITH HIV/AIDS*

Weissman, G. and Brown, V. 1996. Drug-Using Women and HIV: Access to Care and Treatment Issues. In A. O'Leary and L.S. Jemmott (Eds.), *Women and AIDS: Coping and Care* (pp. 109-121). New York: Plenum Press

Weitz, R. 1990. Living with the Stigma of AIDS. *Qualitative Sociology* 13:23-38.

Weitz, R. 1991. *Life with AIDS.* New Brunswick: Rutgers University Press.

Weitz, R. 1993. Powerlessness, Invisibility, and the Lives of Women with HIV Disease. In G.L. Albrecht and R. Zimmerman (Eds.), *Advances in Medical Sociology: The Social and Behavioral Aspects of AIDS* (pp. 101-121). Greenwich, CT: JAI Press.

Wells, D.V.B. and Jackson, J.F. 1992. HIV and Chemically Dependent Women: Recommendations for Appropriate Health Care and Drug Treatment Services. *The International Journal of the Addictions* 27:571-585.

Wiener, L.S. 1991. Women and Human Immunodeficiency Virus: A Historical and Personal Psychosocial Perspective. *Social Work* 36:375-378.

Wight, R.G., LeBlanc, A.J., and Aneshensel, C.S. 1995. Support Service Use by Persons with AIDS and their Caregivers. *AIDS Care* 7:509-520.

Wight, R.G., LeBlanc, A.J., and Aneshensel, C.S. 1998. AIDS Caregiving and Health Among Midlife and Older Women. *Health Psychology* 17:130-137.

Williams, G. 1984. The Genesis of Chronic Illness: Narrative Re-Construction. *Sociology of Health and Illness* 6:175-200. Belmont: Wadsworth.

Williams, J.K. 1995. Afro-American Women Living with HIV Infection: Special Therapeutic Interventions for a Growing Population. *Social Work in Health Care* 21:41-53.

Wilson, J. 1993. Women As Carers, Scotland. In M. Berer (Ed.), *Women and HIV/AIDS: An International Resource Book* (pp. 287-288). London: Pandora Press.

Woods, T.E., Antoni, M.H., Ironson, G.H., and Kling, D.W. 1999. Religiosity Is Associated with Affective Status in Symptomatic HIV-Infected African-American Women. *Journal of Health Psychology* 4:317-326.

Wright, F. 1983. Single Careers: Employment, Housework, and Caring. In J. Finch and D. Groves (Eds.), *A Labour of Love: Women, Work, and Caring* (pp. 89-105). Boston: Routledge and Kegan Paul.

Wyche, K.F. 1998. Let Me Suffer So My Kids Won't: African-American Mothers Living with HIV/AIDS. In C.G. Coll, J.L. Surrey, and K. Weingarten (Eds.), *Mothering Against the Odds: Diverse Voices of Contemporary Mothers* (pp. 173-189). New York: Guilford Press.

Young, R. and Kahana, E. 1989. Specifying Caregiver Outcomes: Gender and the Relationship Aspects of Caregiver Strain. *The Gerontologist* 29:660-666.

Zarit, S.H., Todd, P.A., and Zarit, J.M. 1986. Subjective Burden of Husbands and Wives As Caregivers: A Longitudinal Study. *The Gerontologist* 26:260-266.

Zierler, S. 1997. Hitting Hard: HIV and Violence. In N. Goldstein and J.L. Manlowe (Eds.), *The Gender Politics of HIV/AIDS: Perspectives on the Pandemic in the United States* (pp. 207-221). New York: New York University Press.

Zierler, S., Cunningham, W.E., Anderson, R., Shapiro, M.F., Nakazono, T., Morton, S., Crystal, S., Stein, M., Turner, B., St. Clair, P., and Bozzette, S.A. 2000. Violence Victimization After HIV Infection in a U.S. Probability Sample of Adult Patients in Primary Care. *American Journal of Public Health* 90:208-215.

Index

Page numbers followed by the letter "t" indicate a table.

WOMEN'S EXPERIENCES WITH HIV/AIDS
Mending Fractured Selves

_____in hardbound at $22.46 (regularly $29.95) (ISBN: 0-7890-1757-1)

_____in softbound at $14.96 (regularly $19.95) (ISBN: 0-7890-1758-X)

Or order online and use Code HEC25 in the shopping cart.